COMPUTERS IN NUCLEAR MEDICINE:
A PRACTICAL APPROACH

COMPUTERS IN NUCLEAR MEDICINE: A PRACTICAL APPROACH

Kai H. Lee, PhD

Nuclear Medicine Section
Department of Radiology
University of Southern California School of Medicine
Los Angeles, California

Published by
The Society of Nuclear Medicine
136 Madison Avenue, New York, NY 10016

The Society of Nuclear Medicine, Inc.
136 Madison Avenue, New York, NY 10016-6760

© 1991 by The Society of Nuclear Medicine, Inc. All rights reserved. This book is protected by copyright. No part of it may be reproduced, stored in a retrieval system, or transmitted, in any form or by any means, electronic, mechanical, photocopying, recording, or otherwise, without the prior written permission of the publisher.

Made in the United States of America

Library of Congress Cataloging in Publication Data

Lee, Kai.
    Computers in nuclear medicine: a practical approach by/Kai Lee
      p. cm.
    Includes bibliographical references and index.
    ISBN 0-932004-36-9: $35.00
    1. Radioisotope scanning—Data processing. 2. Image processing.
I. Title.
    [DNLM: 1. Computers. 2. Nuclear Medicine. WN 26.5 L748c]
RC78.7.R4L44 1991
616.07' 575' 0285—dc20
DNLM/DLC
for Library of Congress   91-4859
                                                                           CIP

PREFACE

The role of computers in nuclear medicine has grown from a research curiosity in the early 1970s to become an indispensible tool of current clinical practice. For example, routine nuclear medicine studies such as multi-gated cardiac studies and emission tomography would have been impossible without computers. However, for many nuclear medicine practitioners, the computer remains an intimidating black box with which they never feel at ease.

This book is written for those who want to acquire a basic understanding on how computers work and the processing techniques used to obtain diagnostic information from radionuclide images. Frankly, we do not need to know the computer inside out before we can start utilizing it to obtain useful clinical information. How many people cared to learn how refrigerators work before they brought one home? Likewise, you do not need to know how an internal combustion engine works before you can drive a car. However, if we have a basic understanding of how computers work, we may not only lessen our "computerphobia," but we may also become much more proficient in devising new studies using the computer and in recognizing artifacts when the computer is misbehaving. By the same token, if a motorist has a basic understanding of the operating principles of automobiles, many road emergencies will not seem as frightening.

With this objective in mind, the text is presented as a simple but thorough introduction to the inner workings of a nuclear medicine computer system — what the hardware components are and how they function individually and in conjunction with each other to accomplish a given task. Learning about the nuts and bolts in a computer is only a small portion of the story. The larger portion requires an understanding of the instructions given to the computer to produce the information needed for patient management. To achieve this aim, an empirical approach has been used to explain the principles behind many common image processing techniques by working with examples and avoiding "heavy duty" mathematics as much as possible. To unify the various topics in previous chapters, I selected two areas of nuclear medicine that require the computer to produce results (i.e., nuclear cardiology and emission computed tomography) to demonstrate how we make use of different computer hardware and image processing techniques.

This book is organized into short chapters with "lighthearted" wording and liberal use of drawings so the reader can leisurely read through highly technical information and see how a complex image analysis system is built from individually simple modules. Topics requiring moderate mathematics are relegated to the Appendices for interested readers. Instead of writing a single chapter on the latest developments in nuclear medicine computing with a number of unrelated topics in it, I chose to intersperse such discussions in relevant places in the text. In this fashion, readers will obtain a good perspective on how some of the current computing problems will be solved in the future. I learned a lot while writing this book. I hope that it also will become a learning tool for readers with no prior knowledge of computers.

Finally, I wish to express my appreciation to Patrick Ford, MD and Christiaan Schiepers, PhD, MD who reviewed the manuscript and provided many helpful suggestions. I would also like to thank my wife, Susanna, for her encouragement during the various stages of writing this book.

TABLE OF CONTENTS

Preface v

CHAPTER 1
FUNCTIONS AND COMPONENTS
OF A COMPUTER SYSTEM
    Introduction 1
    Basic Structures of a Computer System 1
    The Central Processing Unit 2
    Performance Rating of the CPU 4
    Memory Unit 7
    What Comprises a Bit? 15
    Conclusions 18

CHAPTER 2
MASS STORAGE DEVICES
    Introduction 21
    Magnetic Disk Storage Devices 22
    A Look Into the Future of Magnetic Disk Technology ... 32
    Optical Disks 34
    Magnetic Tape Drives 37
    Conclusions 42

CHAPTER 3
INPUT AND OUTPUT DEVICES
    Introduction 43
    Input Devices 43
    Output Devices 50
    Printers 60
    Conclusions 65
    Suggested Readings 65

CHAPTER 4
COMPUTER SOFTWARE
    Introduction 67
    Types of Computer Software 68
    Operating System 69

Programming Software 74
Conclusions 80
Suggested Readings 86

CHAPTER 5
NUCLEAR MEDICINE IMAGE ACQUISITION METHODS

Introduction 87
Methods of Data Acquisition 87
Frame-Mode Acquisition 88
Byte-Mode Versus Word-Mode Acquisition 93
Dynamic Frame-Mode Acquisition 95
Multiple-Gated and List-Mode Acquisition 97
Conclusion 98
Suggested Readings 98

CHAPTER 6
METHODS OF QUALITATIVE IMAGE ANALYSIS

Introduction 99
Image Enhancement 99
Convolution Methods of Image Enhancement 100
Fourier Methods of Image Enhancement 107
Point Processing Operations 113
Frame Processing Operations 123
Geometric Operations 123
Conclusion 124
Suggested Readings 125

CHAPTER 7
QUANTITATIVE IMAGE ANALYSIS

Introduction 127
Creating ROIs 128
Curve Generation and Analysis 134
Conclusion 145

CHAPTER 8
NUCLEAR CARDIOLOGY

Introduction 147
Methods of Data Acquisition 148
Analysis of Multiple-Gated Blood-Pool Images 158

CONTENTS

Quantitative Data Analysis............................. 164
First-Pass Cardiac Studies............................. 176
Methods of Data Reformatting for First-Pass Studies......... 178
Planar Quantification of Myocardial Perfusion............. 185
Conclusion... 187
Suggested Readings................................... 188

CHAPTER 9
SINGLE-PHOTON EMISSION
COMPUTED TOMOGRAPHY
    Introduction....................................... 189
    Instrumentation System Description.................. 190
    Mathematics of Transverse Image Reconstruction....... 193
    Physical Factors Affecting the Quality of SPECT Images.. 207
    Quality Assurance of the SPECT System.............. 220
    Conclusion.. 226
    Suggested Readings................................ 227

CHAPTER 10
AN ALL-DIGITAL NUCLEAR
MEDICINE DEPARTMENT
Introdution.. 229
Communication Networks............................. 230
Local Area Network Topology......................... 233
An Overview of PACS................................. 237
Conclusion... 240
Suggested Readings................................... 241

CHAPTER 11
CRITERIA FOR THE SELECTION OF
A NUCLEAR MEDICINE COMPUTER
    Introduction 243
    Software... 244
    User Support..................................... 248
    Measurement of User-Friendliness................... 249
    Image Display.................................... 250
    Hardware.. 251
    Reliability and Service Support..................... 253
    Conclusion....................................... 253
    Suggested Reading................................ 254

APPENDIX A
Digital Number Systems 255

APPENDIX B
How Successive Approximation of
Analog-to-Digital Converters Work 259

APPENDIX C
A Numerical Example of Fourier Transform 263

APPENDIX D
Color Scans 271

INDEX 275

CHAPTER

1

FUNCTIONS AND COMPONENTS OF A COMPUTER SYSTEM

INTRODUCTION

Computers are similar to many sophisticated devices, which on the surface, may appear hopelessly complicated. Once the computer is broken down into its principal components and the primary functions of each module is described, the computer system as a whole is not so mysterious. This chapter will introduce to the uninitiated reader the basic building blocks of a typical computer system, how each component works, and why we need it.

BASIC STRUCTURES OF A COMPUTER SYSTEM

A computer is an electronic black box capable of receiving, storing, manipulating, and communicating information. All the nuts and bolts and electronic widgets inside the awe-inspiring black box are called hardware and are classified into four major categories:

1. Central processing unit.
2. Memory unit.
3. Mass storage devices.
4. Input and output devices.

An overview diagram of these four major functional units is shown in Figure 1-1. Once these four intertwined units are initiated by a set of instructions (i.e., a computer program), the computer system

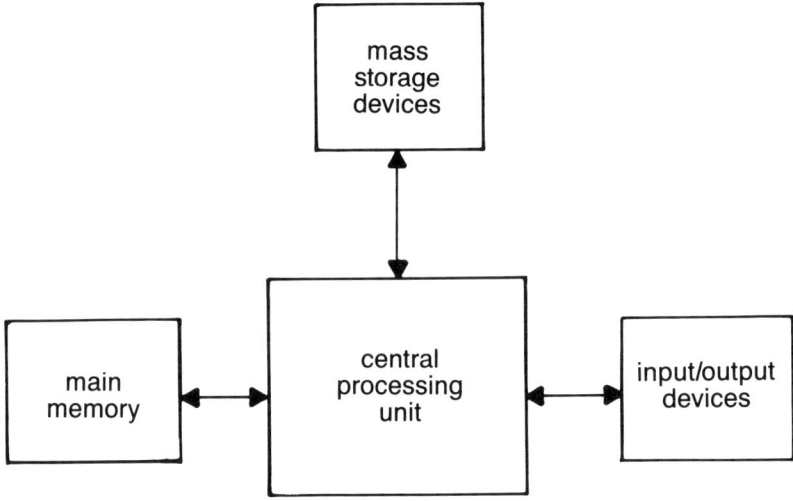

FIGURE 1-1 The basic building blocks of a computer system.

will faithfully execute the instructions one at a time automatically without further human interventions.

This type of system design is known as von Neumann architecture, after the design principles published in 1945 by the mathematician John von Neumann. Basically, computers designed with the von Neumann principles utilize: (1) a central processing unit (CPU) to perform computations and regulate the system operations, (2) a memory unit to hold data and program instructions, and (3) input/output devices to communicate information into and out of the computer. Such a machine works with binary numbers and performs one instruction at a time in sequence.

THE CENTRAL PROCESSING UNIT

The heart of a computer system is the CPU, which not only performs arithmetic and logic functions but also coordinates the communication of information between the different hardware components and directs the sequence of operations of the entire computer system. These functions are handled by two major sub-units within the CPU: the control unit and the arithmetic and logic unit (ALU).

Control Unit

The control unit is designed to recognize a set of coded electronic pulses, also known as instruction sets, that tells it to perform specific functions. When the computer is requested to perform a task, the control unit will direct and supervise all operations of the system components in an order exactly as specified in the sequences of instruction codes. It reads one instruction at a time, starting at the beginning of the sequence of instruction codes stored in the CPU memory, and interprets each one. It then sends signals to trigger the appropriate components in the computer system to perform the required operation. When the execution of the current instruction is completed, the control unit reads the next instruction, interprets its meaning, and passes control signals to other components in the computer system to perform the next operation. Thus, the control unit coordinates all operations in the entire computer system. The control unit takes command of the input/output devices, the arithmetic and logic operations, and the transfer of data to and from storage. It directs the sequence of operations to be performed on the data, but performs no actual processing operations on the data. The data manipulation functions are delegated by the control unit to other sub-units in the system.

Arithmetic and Logic Unit

The ALU is the number cruncher and is responsible for all arithmetic and logic operations on the input data. Although the ALU can be designed to perform a variety of exotic mathematical and logical operations, the four fundamental arithmetic operations (addition, subtraction, multiplication, and division) are the "bread and butter" operations in all computer systems. It should be noted that the ALU will add, subtract, or perform whatever operation the control unit directs. To avoid the "garbage in garbage out syndrome," the control unit not only needs to supply the ALU with all the proper data, but also supply it in the correct sequence.

PERFORMANCE RATING OF THE CPU

The performance of the CPU has to be rated on the basis of a number of parameters. However, speed is used more than any other parameter as the index of computer power. This is understandable considering the constant aim toward increasing computer speed. CPU speed generally is quoted in the commercial literature by either the clock rate or the number of instructions that the CPU can execute in a second.

In every CPU, there is a clock that sends out precisely timed pulses for as long as the machine is running. The control unit monitors these timing pulses and uses them to synchronize the operations in the CPU. The shortest interval between each tick of the clock is determined by the time required for the pulse to travel the longest path within the CPU. Thus, one way to increase CPU speed is to miniaturize the electronic components to reduce travel distance. The top speed of the current micro-processors is about 50 MHz (50 megahertz or 50 million ticks per second), but CPUs running at 40, 32, 24, 16, 12, and 8 MHz are also in daily use.

Keep in mind, however, that a CPU running at 32 MHz does not necessarily process data twice as fast as a 16 MHz CPU, nor four times as fast as an 8 MHz CPU. The CPU with a faster clock will complete its assigned tasks sooner than one with a slower clock, but the rate at which the CPU gets its job done is not always directly proportional to the clock rate.

The other common method for specifying CPU speed is to calculate how many million instructions per second (Mips) the CPU can finish. Of course, when we measure the processing speed of the CPU in terms of Mips, we must also specify the type of instructions used in making the benchmark. However, we can get a feel for the relative speed of different classes of computers without dwelling on the details of the test instructions. At the time of this writing, the common general-purpose mini- and micro-computers work in a range between one to several Mips; RISC workstations run between 10 to 40 Mips; super-mini and mainframe computers operate from several tens to over 100 Mips; while supercomputers perform at 200 Mips and higher.

We have witnessed quantum leaps in computing speeds when we changed our machines from mechanical devices to electronic vacuum tubes, from vacuum tubes to transistors, and from transistors to integrated circuits. In addition to finding ways to build swifter hardware, progress is being made to build faster computers using non-traditional designs, such as reduced-instruction set computers (RISC) architecture and parallel architecture.

Reduced Instruction Set Computers

By one definition, a computer's architecture is a set of instructions built into the hardware for data handling and program executions. With the ever decreasing size of integrated circuits, more and more instructions can be hard-wired into one silicon chip. This type of computer architecture is known as complex instruction set computers (CISC). The advantage of having a large number of instructions built into the hardware is that many complicated operations can be carried out in a few steps. However, studies have found that less than 20% of the hundreds of instructions available in the CISC units were actually used in the vast majority of computing applications. Much of the built-in instructions were excess baggage, resulting in increased design and manufacturing costs and slowing of processing speed.

The objective of RISC architecture is to increase the efficiency of the CPU by optimizing the use of a small set of simple instructions in the hardware. During program execution, a number of simple instructions are called upon to perform the equivalent of one complex instruction. RISC wins the speed race because it can easily synchronize the execution of a number of simple instructions in an assembly-line fashion. For example, one instruction can be executed, while the next instruction is being translated to machine codes, and the one after that is being retrieved from the memory. This assembly-line technique in which parts of different instructions are carried out simultaneously is called *pipelining*. Due to the efficiency of the assembly-line and the fast execution of simple instructions, the overall gain in speed is more than compensated for the extra number of required steps. Since 1989, the growth of RISC-based computers for graphics and image processing has been phenomenal. The intense competition among computer manufacturers is evidenced not only by the rapid decline of system cost, but by announcements of new RISC systems every three to four months. This trend is likely to continue throughout the early 1990s.

The success of RISC will have a significant impact on nuclear medicine image processing. The computations involved in the processing of nuclear medicine images, such as SPECT and three-dimensional image reconstruction, are simple but time-comsuming because each computation is repeated thousands of times. This is precisely RISC's claim—execution of simple instructions at lightning speed. When nuclear medicine imaging software is implemented on RISC systems, many analyses that currently could not be done because of unacceptably long computation time will become practical.

Parallel Processing

As described above, the control unit divides a job into a number of smaller tasks and then sequentially assigns each task to be completed by different sub-units in the CPU. This means that at any given time parts of the CPU are idle while one task is being completed. While significant speeds have been gained by putting the idle elements to work, today's super-computers performing at 200 to 500 Mips may be already approaching the theoretical bound of about 3 billion instructions per second for computers built based on the von Neumann architecture.

Unlike the von Neumann architecture, which uses a CPU to carry out its work sequentially, a parallel computer distributes the work to a multiple number of processing units, called nodes. Each node is a self-sufficient computer with its own CPU and memory. By permitting a number of processors to work on different parts of a problem simultaneously, speed in trillions of instructions per second are theoretically possible.

One example of parallel architecture that has produced much excitement is the *hypercube design* in which the computer is thought of as a cube with a node at each corner. The number of nodes in the computer is the dimension of the hypercube. Within the hypercube, each node works independently with its own data and communicates with each other while executing program instructions. At the completion of the task, partial results from each node are combined to produce the final output. Hypercubes have been built using tens and even hundreds of CPUs that work on different parts of a program simultaneously.

Hypercube computers are best suited to solve problems that can be processed independently in small parts. Delays do occur when one node requires information that is being processed in another node. Fortunately, image processing lends itself very well for parallel computing because each node can work independently on data for different parts of the image, or different data for the same image, and one node can be instructed to form the final composite image using results from the other nodes.

Geologists have used parallel computers with great success to analyze the voluminous seismic data obtained from oil field explorations and to map the earth's resources using satellite data. Unfortunately, parallel computers are too expensive for nuclear medicine image processing at the present time. However, in the 1960s who would have thought that laptop computers the size of a notebook would be more powerful that those in a freezing computing center.

MEMORY UNIT

The memory unit has been called the CPU memory, the main memory, and primary storage. The CPU memory is the most frequently quoted item, and is perhaps the most mysterious unit to the beginner. The CPU memory consists of several hundred thousand and, commonly millions, of storage elements, much like the dazzling array of mail boxes in a post office. Each memory element (mail box) is assigned an address (P.O. box number), which enables the control unit to find a particular element and either write data into or read data from it. In computer jargon, a storage element is called a *memory location* (mail box) with a *memory address* (P.O. box number).

The computer memory is used to hold a variety of information. Some storage locations in the memory are reserved for storing program instructions, some contain data, and some are used to hold processing results. The size of each memory location and the number of locations determine how many instructions can be kept in the computer and how sophisticated these operations can be. An analogous situation occurs in a post office where the greater the number of mail boxes available and the larger the size of each box, the greater the amount of mail the post office can hold. This is one of the reasons why the capability of a computer system can often be inferred from its memory size.

The amount of memory in a computer is quantified in units of *bytes*. In the 1970s, computer memory was expensive and there was a limitation on the number of memory addresses that a CPU could track. A typical nuclear medicine computer used then contained between 65,536 bytes (64 KB) to 131,072 bytes (128 KB) of memory — the prefix kilo or K stands for 1,024 (2^{10}) not 1,000 (10^3). Due to the reduced cost of computer memory and the availability of more powerful CPUs, the CPU memory was increased to between 256 KB to 1 MB (1 million bytes or 1,048,576 bytes) by the mid-1980s and undoubtedly will retain tens of megabytes in the 1990s.

A Word on Bits and Bytes

All computers (super, mainframe, mini-, and micro-computers) share one common feature: they all use the binary system to represent numbers and non-numeric characters such as the alphabet. Readers who are "rusty" on binary arithmetic may review the fundamentals of binary arithmetic in Appendix A. The main reason for the universal use of binary digits to represent the information in computers is the ease with which binary digits can be represented by simple magnetic and electrical devices.

The term binary digit is used so frequently that it has been given an acronym, *bit*. A bit is the most fundamental unit of information in a computer. It is allowed to have a value of only zero or one. Because a bit carries so little information, a group of eight bits were strung together to form one larger unit of information known as a *byte*. The group of eight bits in a byte can have 256 different combinations of zeroes and ones, which is far greater than the two possible combinations with only one bit. For example, one byte is adequate to represent all the characters found on the keyboard of a computer, i.e., the upper and lower case letters, numbers, punctuation marks and special symbols.

The term *word* is confusing at times to the novice. A computer word is a unit of information processed by the CPU at one time. In the 1970s, a large number of mini-computers utilized a sequence

FUNCTIONS AND COMPONENTS

of 16 bits, instead of 8 bits, as a primary unit of information. People working with these computers used the term word to mean 16 bits or 2 bytes. The ambiguity arises because many of the minicomputers still in use at that time and the burgeoning microcomputers were working in 8-bit units. For this class of computers, a word carried 8 bits or 1 byte, and users of the 8-bit computers were using the terms word and byte interchangeably. The point to remember is that a word is a group of bits processed together by the CPU as one basic unit of information that can have any number of bits in it. In order to reduce the confusion, a convention was evolved to describe the amount of CPU memory in bytes. The meaning of word was standardized to denote 16 bits, The relationship between a bit, a byte, and a word is shown in Figure 1-2.

With the rapid developments in computer technology, the newer CPUs were able to handle 32 bits and 64 bits in a single operation. New terms had to be invented to quantify larger units of information. The term *long-word* was invented to mean a chunk of 32 bits, *quad-word* to mean 64 bits, and *octa-word* to mean 128 bits. However, the terms long-word, quad-word, and octa-word are not standard.

If the relationhip between bits, bytes and words is confusing, try quantifying CPU memory size in *nibbles*! One nibble is half of

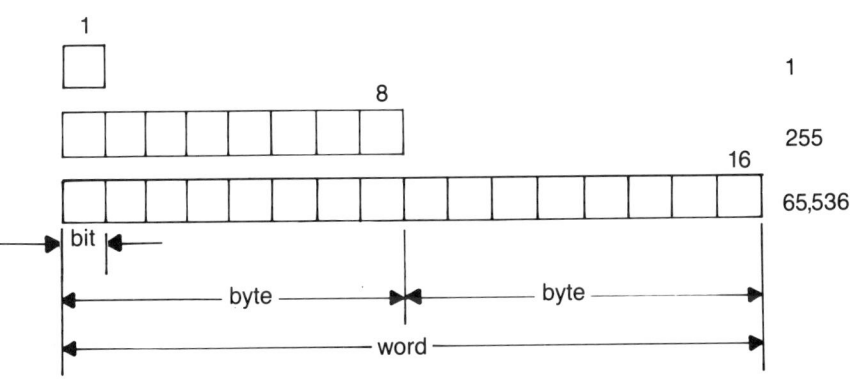

FIGURE 1-2 One bit is one binary digit that can have a numerical value of either zero or one. One byte is a string of eight bits, and one word equals 2 bytes or 16 bits.

a byte or 4 bits. In the "medieval" time of computers, information was also grouped in "crumbs," with one crumb equaling two bits. Fortunately, computers that work on crumbs and nibbles are only found in museums.

Word-length

The number of bits that the computer can handle as a whole is quantified by the term *word-length*. The word-length is a characteristic of the CPU. It varies from 8 bits in computers of 1960s vintage to 64 bits in mainframe computers. If a computer is described as a 32-bit computer, this means that the computer is capable of processing a group of 32 bits in one operation. The trend in computer development has been to design computers with longer and longer word-length. With a longer word-length, more information can be processed in each computer operation. One byte, for example, is sufficient to represent one letter of the English alphabet or one special symbol, such as #, +, =, or $. Since one of the eight bits in a byte is needed to represent either a + or − sign, the maximum absolute value that one byte can hold is 127 ($2^7 - 1$). If the computer has a 16-bit word-length, two letters can be stored in one memory location and the largest absolute value that can be kept in one location is 32,767 ($2^{15} - 1$). In addition, computations can be carried out with greater precision if more bits are available to represent the number of digits after the decimal point.

Word-length also affects the amount of memory that the computer system can have. Remember that the CPU communicates with a memory location in the memory unit by first looking up its memory address. For an 8-bit CPU there can be only 256 available addresses ($2^8 = 256$), and only 65,536 available addresses ($2^{16} = 65,536$) for a 16-bit CPU. In the 1960s and 1970s, computer manufacturers had to devise a cumbersome scheme for an 8-bit CPU to manage 64 kilobytes of memory and 1 mega-byte for a 16-bit CPU. With a 32-bit CPU, widely available in the late 1980s, the computer can support up to 4 gigabytes (4 billion bytes, $2^{32} = 4,294,967,296$) of memory without resorting to tricky memory management schemes.

The advantage of longer word-length goes beyond greater storage capacity in the memory. The processing speed of the computer can also be increased with a longer word-length. As previously discussed, the computer handles a group of bits at a time. Since more information can be stored in 32 bits, a 32-bit computer will take fewer steps than a 16-bit computer to process the same amount of data, thus reducing processing time.

Random Access Memory

One important characteristic of the CPU memory is that each byte of memory has an unique address. The CPU can gain access to any memory location directly without having to step through other intermediate addresses. The time required to reach a randomly selected address in the CPU memory is the same regardless of its location in the memory. This type of memory is called random access memory (RAM), which has a second important feature. Data or program instructions can be read from or written to the RAM at will by the user. The CPU can read the contents of a particular byte of memory by sending a signal to the appropriate address, or it can write information to the memory location and replace the contents already stored there. Because it is flexible, the user can alter the program instructions, update data, or retrieve information in the RAM rapidly. The purpose of the RAM is to provide a temporary storage for program instructions and data. The contents in the RAM continually change as program execution progresses.

Read-Only Memory

Program instructions or data that do not require frequent alterations but need to be accessed very quickly are usually kept in a read only memory (ROM). Every computer has one or more ROMs. Contents in the ROM can be read but cannot be changed by the user. One use of the ROM is in the computer's start-up procedure called *bootstrapping*, or booting for short. When we turn on the computer's power switch, the surge of electricity activates the system's clock which in turn triggers a signal to clear the memory and reset all the circuits to the startup conditions. On the next trigger of the clock, the CPU is directed to execute the first of a series of instructions stored in the ROM. As the clock pulses on, thousands of instructions stored in the ROM, and some on an external disk, will be executed one by one until the computer is ready for user input.

This automatic start-up procedure is called bootstrapping because the computer in effect pulls itself up by its own bootstrap.

The program instructions or data that were put into the ROM are permanent in the computer system. When the power to the computer is turned off, nothing is lost from the ROM. On the other hand, every power outage will erase all information from the RAM. In order to alter the contents in a ROM, the ROM has to be removed from the computer and replaced by another with an updated content. For this reason, ROM is called *firmware*. The concept to keep in mind is that the contents in a ROM are permanent and can only be changed by a special device.

Cache Memory

Cache memory is a small, high speed memory buffer between the CPU and the main memory, as shown in Figure 1-3. Cache memory works on the principle that the CPU has a high probability in the near future to use the information on which it is currently working. A cache memory is designed to ensure that when such information is needed, the CPU can obtain it quickly from the cache, without having to go to the slower main memory. Given the millions of bytes of memory required for modern computing, micro-electronic switches that are slower but cheaper than those in the CPU were used to construct the memory chips. After issuing a request for information from the memory, the CPU has to pause for the information to arrive.

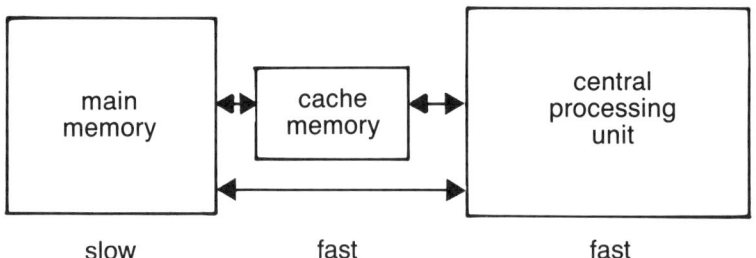

FIGURE 1-3 A typical read cycle in a system with cache memory. The high-speed CPU first looks into its high-speed cache memory to see if the desired data are there. If not, it then sits and waits for the slower main memory to transfer the data.

The CPU is said to be in a *wait-state* while it is waiting for the information to be transferred from the slower memory unit. By placing the frequently used data and instructions in the cache memory, the CPU takes only about one-tenth the amount of time that otherwise would be needed to obtain data from the main memory. Clearly, the larger the cache, the better the system performance. Unfortunately, cache is like cash; no one seems to have too much, and everyone is constantly short of it. Due to the expense of high speed memory, cache memory size is commonly about 64 KB and rarely exceeds 256 KB. Therefore, designers of cache memory have to make difficult decisions on the strategies used to retrieve and update information in the cache.

Buffer Memory

Buffer memory is a special type of RAM used to bridge the differences in rate of data flow when transferring data between the CPU and its peripheral devices. A computer always includes a number of peripheral devices connected to the CPU to form a functional system. However, most peripheral devices, especially those used for data input and output, complete their assigned tasks at speeds much slower than the CPU. Inefficient use of the computer becomes obvious if the CPU must intermittently pause for input and output operations to be completed and cannot do anything else during these pauses. Let us say we want the computer to print out the names and addresses of a list of patients on a paper printer. The CPU can transfer the data from the memory at thousands of characters per second, while an average printer may put out only about 200 characters per second. This means that the CPU is forced to slow down to keep pace with the slower printer. The slow paper printer thus becomes the bottleneck of the entire computer operation.

The buffer memory acts as an intermediate holding area for data coming in from the CPU at a high speed and going out at a much slower pace, as shown in Figure 1-4. The buffer memory is located outside the CPU memory and is invariably linked to a peripheral device. If a paper printer in the above example is buffered, the buffer memory first receives and stores the names and addresses of patients sent out from the CPU at high speed. After the CPU completes this task in a hurry, it continues on to perform other duties

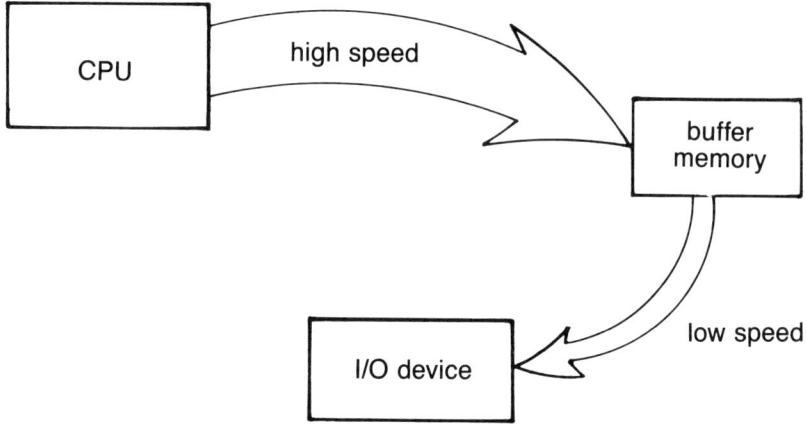

FIGURE 1-4 The buffer memory serves as the temporary holding area for data communication with the CPU at high speed and the I/O devices at a much slower speed.

while the printer is slowly making an imprint on paper of the data stored in the buffer.

To illustrate further, a buffer memory is used in nearly all nuclear medicine computer systems in connection with the acquisition and display of radionuclide images from a gamma camera. It may take several minutes to accumulate a sufficient number of counts for a radionuclide image. If the input device responsible for acquiring counts from the gamma camera were buffered, the input data would be instructed by the CPU to assemble in the buffer memory, while other tasks could be taking place in the CPU in the mean time. After the required number of counts for an image had been accumulated, data in the buffer memory would then be transferred to the CPU memory for processing in a small fraction of the time that would be required to read in the data directly from the gamma camera.

As another example, the display unit of the nuclear medicine computer system consists of a video display monitor, a video display controller, and a display memory (also known as the frame buffer). In order to maintain a flicker-free image on the video monitor, the screen must be refreshed at least 30 or more times a second. If the CPU must be called upon to repetitively refresh the video display, hardly anything else can be done by the CPU whenever an image is shown on the screen. By placing a video display memory or frame buffer between the CPU and the video display, the matrix of data making up the video image is transferred to the buffer memory by the CPU in one operation. Once the transfer is completed, the display controller simply reads the successive bytes of data from the frame buffer and converts the zeroes and ones into the corresponding electrical signals. The signals are then sent to the video display monitor, producing an image with the appropriate colors and intensities. The display controller repeats this process of converting the contents of the frame buffer to video signals over and over again to maintain a steady image. Meanwhile, the CPU is freed from this repetitive chore and can be utilized maximally to perform other tasks.

If a number of buffer memories are connected to a computer system, data input, output, and processing can then occur simultaneously. For example, data coming from a gamma camera could be filling the acquisition buffer, processing of other image data could be taking place in the CPU, and the display of a buffered image could occur on another display station all at the same time. Thus, a buffer memory prevents the slow input and output operations from dragging down the operating efficiency of the CPU. Also, this buffer memory extends the data storage capacity of the computer.

WHAT COMPRISES A BIT?

Semiconductor Memory

Current computer memories are predominantly made of metal oxide semiconductors (MOS). MOS memories consist of many hundred thousand, and now millions, of micro-switches fabricated in a tiny silicon chip. Each micro-switch controlled circuit in the chip represents one bit. As shown in Figure 1-5, we can arbitrarily assign the conducting conditions equivalent to 1 and the off condition equivalent to 0. The on or off condition of a circuit therefore represents one bit of information. The common number of bits making up a memory chip is 1-megabit; the 4-megabit memory chips are used on the high performance computers.

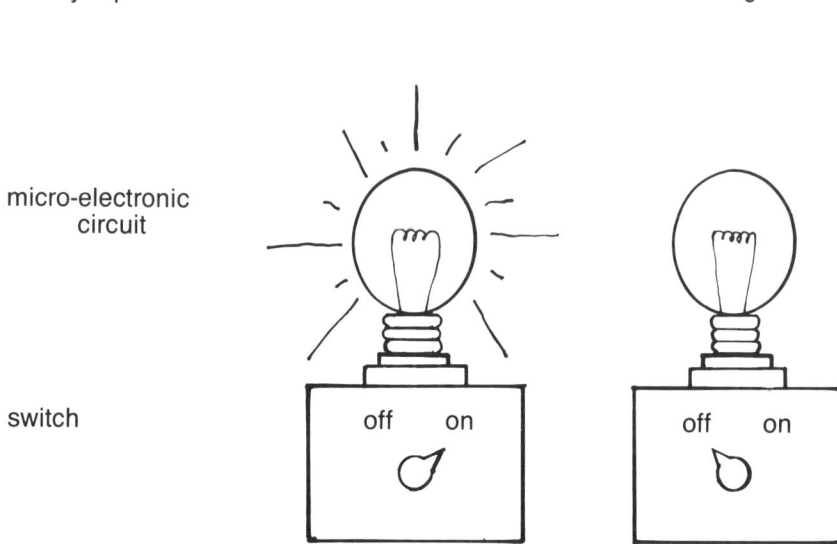

FIGURE 1-5 MOS memory uses one micro-electronic circuit to represent one bit. Information is coded in the MOS memory by switching groups of circuits to a combination of "On" and "Off" pattern.

The major advantages of MOS memories are:

1. Compactness. Thousands of bytes can be packaged into a silicon chip about the size of a finger nail.
2. Low manufacturing cost for semi-conductors, which continues to drop.
3. They consume little electric power.
4. Rapid read/write operations.

Unfortunately, MOS memories are vulnerable to power fluctuations. MOS memories require a stable, uninterrupted supply of electrical power because information in a memory chip is coded by the presence or absence of electrical charge in each micro-circuit. If there is a power outage or large power fluctuation, the pattern of "On" and "Off" circuits in the chip is altered and the stored information is either erased completely or becomes nonsensical.

Core Memory

An older type of RAM uses magnetic cores, which are used only sparingly in the modern computers. It is instructional, however, to review the operating principles of magnetic cores to show how the binary number system is used to represent information in the computer. A magnetic core is a doughnut-shaped piece of ferrite material that can be easily magnetized. Figure 1-6 shows a wire passing through the core. An electric current passing through the wire will induce a magnetic field in the ferrite core. The direction of the magnetic field follows the right-hand rule. If the current passes from the left to the right, a magnetic field is induced in the core in the counter-clockwise direction. If the current reverses its direction, the magnetic field is induced in the clockwise direction. So the direction of the core magnetic field can be easily changed by switching an electric current through the wire in the opposite direction. By arbitrarily assigning the clockwise direction of the magnetic field to represent 0 and the counter-clockwise direction to represent 1, a core can be used to represent one bit of information. Eight of these cores strung together becomes one byte. A computer's core memory is made up of thousands of these cores arranged in an orderly fashion.

One distinct characteristic of core memory is that the core remains magnetized indefinitely in the direction that was last set, until a current is deliberately sent through the wire in the reverse direction. Unlike MOS memories, which require a continuous power supply, core memories remain magnetized in the same direction even

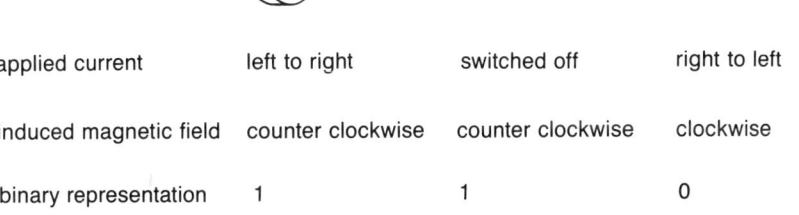

applied current	left to right	switched off	right to left
induced magnetic field	counter clockwise	counter clockwise	clockwise
binary representation	1	1	0

FIGURE 1-6 A bit in the core memory is an iron ring with a wire passing through it. The direction of the magnetic field induced in the iron ring by the applied current determines the binary value of the bit.

after the induction current is removed. Because information stored in the core memory remains unchanged, even after power failure, core memory is called non-volatile memory.

One of the disadvantages of core memory is that it is slower than MOS memory. While a read or write operation in MOS memory can be done in a few tenths of a microsecond, the same operation in core memory takes from one to several microseconds. A second disadvantage is that core memory occupies more space than MOS memory. Although the size of one core is less than one-tenth the size of a dime, hundreds of thousands of these cores collected in one place is quite bulky. A third disadvantage is that more power is required not only to put information into the core, but to keep the cores and its support circuitry cool as well. Do you still remember the cold you got after taking a tour of a refrigerated computer center? Another reason why core memory has fallen from favor is that the manufacturing cost of core memory is higher than that of MOS memory.

Memory of the Future

The ideal memory for a computer must be *inexpensive*, small in size, able to change quickly between the on and off states, and not require special cooling. Of the many proposed memory devices, those made from gallium arsenide pose the greatest immediate threat to the dominance of silicon technology. Room temperature superconductors and optical memories are no longer limited to science fiction movies only. Unfortunately, it is beyond the scope of this primer to survey these forefronts of computer memory devices.

CONCLUSION

The two most closely knitted components of a computer system, the CPU and the memory, have been discussed. Two developments in the 1980s will result in increased preformance of nuclear medicine computers in the 1990s: advancements in the fabrication technique of very large scale integrated (VLSI) circuits that enable several million bits of memory to be built into an area the size of the thumb and the development of 32-bit micro-processors. These 32-bit CPUs not only execute instructions hundreds of times faster than the 16-bit mini-computers, they can also maintain 4 billion bytes (4 GB) of memory and are able to switch rapidly between programs stored in different parts of the CPU memory. The switching takes place so quickly that the user thinks that he has full control of the computer to do several tasks simultaneously. Actually, the CPU is executing pieces of one program and switches rapidly back and forth to execute other programs. This type of computer operation, called multitasking, will be discussed in greater detail in Chapter 4.

With these two technologic advances, the average nuclear medicine computer in the 1990s will carry several megabytes of CPU memory and will be able to perform concurrent operations that are impossible with the current generation of computers. Although the CPU and the memory are the critical components of the computer, we need many other devices, such as disk drives and display monitors, to form a functional computer, store data and program instructions, and show the results to the user. In the next two chapters some of the peripheral devices essential to a nuclear medicine image processing system are discussed.

CHAPTER

2

MASS STORAGE DEVICES

INTRODUCTION

The CPU memory is used for temporary storage of data, program instructions, and computation results. In every computer, the amount of space required for the data and program library far exceeds the capacity of the CPU memory. In such cases, data and programs not currently in use are stored in auxiliary mass storage devices where they can be retrieved when needed.

There are two types of auxiliary mass storage devices— direct access and sequential access storage devices. With a direct access storage device, such as magnetic or optical disk drives, data can be located directly according to its address without scanning through other data. Sequential storage devices such as magnetic tapes and punched cards store information one after another in series. To retrieve a piece of information in the middle of the magnetic tape or stack of cards, all the data ahead of it must be read first. Because the access speed of a disk drive is so much faster than that of a tape drive, virtually every computer employs one or more magnetic disks as the *on-line* mass storage device. However, the ease of changing information on the disk can also be a nightmare to the user. If there is any malfunction in the disk drive, an error in the program or a lapse in the user's alertness, all the programs and patient data can be erased in a fraction of a second. Therefore, it is of utmost importance to periodically copy the information on the disk onto another disk or on magnetic tape as insurance against accidental losses. Since the cost per bit of information stored on magnetic tape is much lower than that of disks, magnetic tapes are widely used *off-line* for backup and archival storage of important information. Optical disks with much larger storage capacity than magnetic disks are available commercially, but this new technology is still in development for use as a substitute for magnetic tapes as the medium for archiving medical images.

MAGNETIC DISK STORAGE DEVICES

There are two common types of magnetic disk storage devices: hard disks and floppy disks. A hard disk is made up of an aluminum platter coated on both surfaces with a material that can be easily magnetized. In the traditional design, the platters were coated with a ferric oxide compound, an exotic scientific term for fine grains of rust in a layer of glue. Recently, the plates were bonded with a thin-film, which is a skinny layer of metal mixture bound electrolytically onto the disk surfaces, much like the "gold" finish on an aluminum picture frame. Thin-films offer much greater resistance to scratches than oxide coatings and allow more data to be packed onto the disk.

Before a new magnetic disk is used, it must first be formatted by the computer. In the formatting process, each surface of the disk is magnetically marked from several hundred to several thousand tracks, much like the tracks on a phonograph record. Unlike the phonograph record's tracks, however, tracks on a disk surface are distinct concentric circles rather than one continuous spiral. Furthermore, each platter of the disk is sub-divided into a number of sectors (like slices of a pie) as shown in Figure 2-1. Data are stored as magnetized spots in the tracks, and addresses are identified by the track number and the sector number in each track. Depending on the number of tracks on the surface, one double-sided disk platter can easily hold 5 MB or more of data. As a comparison, there is only about 8 MB or less of CPU memory in a modern nuclear medicine computer. A 20-Mb disk is much too small by today's standard, but it still can hold as many as 2,000 images of 64 x 64 pixels and 16 bits deep. This amount of data is far more than the CPU memory can hold. Because information stored on disk, whether images or program instructions, can be conveniently brought into the CPU memory when it is needed, some sophisticated computers can use the disk space as an extension of the CPU memory. The term *virtual memory* is used to describe those memory addresses located on the disk.

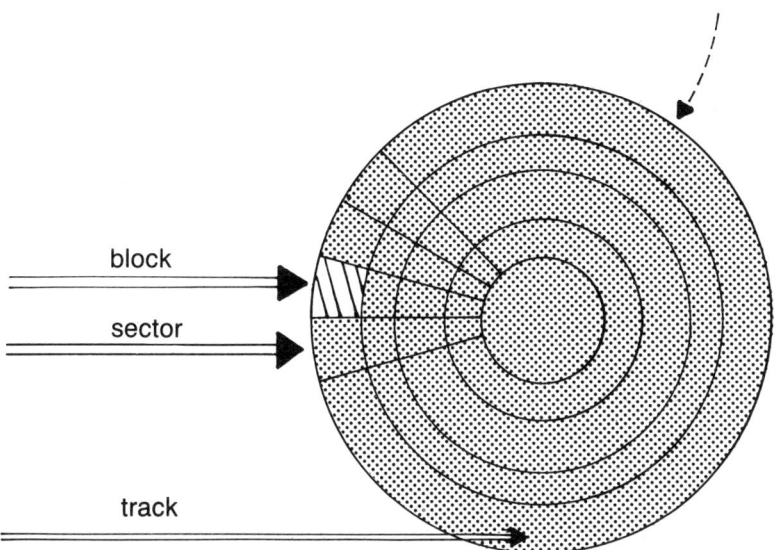

FIGURE 2-1 During formatting, the surface of the disk is divided into concentric tracks and sliced into sectors. The part of the track that lies between the boundaries of two sectors is called a block. Information on the disk is indexed according to the track and sector numbers written each data set.

When a disk is used, it is mounted on the spindle of the disk drive, which turns the disk to about 3600 rpm. To perform read/write operations, a read/write head is provided for each disk surface. When requested to read or write an image on the disk, for example, the access arm on which the head is mounted moves back and forth along a radius of the disk searching for the location of the image. Once the access arm has found the image address, data transfer begins. A read/write operation on the disk of a 64 x 64 image may take approximately 100 to 300 milliseconds to complete. In comparison, the time required for the same read/write operation in the CPU memory only takes about 5 to 10 milliseconds. Thus, the disk extends the storage capacity of the computer at the expense of a reduced speed.

In order to expedite the read/write operations and to achieve a high storage density, the magnetic heads are kept very close to the disk surface, typically in the neighborhood of a few microinches. The distance of separation between the disk and the head, as shown in Figure 2-2, shows that cigarette smoke particles, hair and finger-

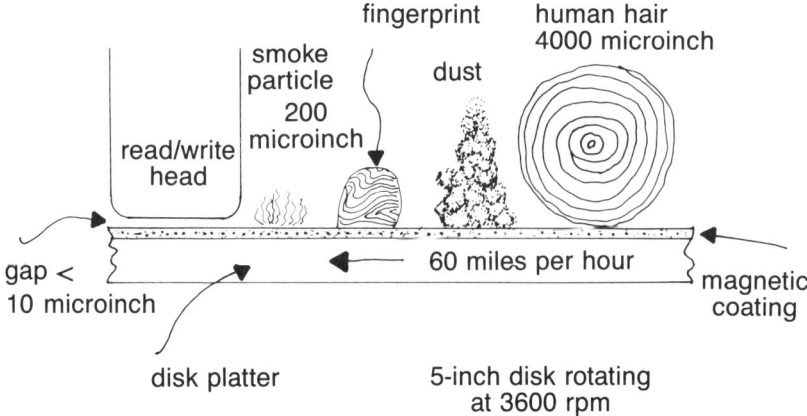

FIGURE 2-2 The common contaminants in a room are at least twenty times bigger than the clearance between the delicate magnetic read/write head and the soft disk surface.

prints are enormous compared to the clearance between the magnetic head and the disk surface.

Normally, with the disk rotating at 3600 rpm, the rushing air between the magnetic head and the disk surface form a soft cushion that floats the head safely at a constant distance above the disk platter. If the head were to collide with a dust particle and crush it on the disk surface moving at such a high speed, the collision could gouge the disk and destroy the head. This disastrous event, resulting in mutual annihilation of the disk and the read/write head, is called a *head crash*. When a head crash occurs, the disk platter and the expensive read/write head must be replaced, and the information stored on the disk is gone forever. For this reason, the air filter on the disk drive must be changed at frequent intervals so that air flowing into the disk chamber is free of harmful contaminants.

Multi-Platter Disk Drives

On many older *disk drives*, one disk platter is permanently mounted in place, while a second removable disk platter (in a plastic casing) is loaded above it on the same spindle; such a removable disk is called a disk cartrdige. Information stored on the top disk can be copied onto the bottom disk and vice versa. This feature is convenient because new patient data or programs can be entered into the computer for processing simply by replacing one disk cartridge with another containing the new information.

An extension of the dual fixed-removable disk concept involves several disk platters combined to form a disk pack, much like the stack of pancakes on your breakfast table each morning. The individual platters on the disk pack, however, cannot be disassembled by the user. The disk pack must be removed from or mounted on the spindle as one unit. This type of disk storage is called *storage module devices* (SMD). A diagram of a disk pack is shown in Figure 2-3.

The multi-platter storage module devices typically have a storage capacity between 80 Mb to 200 Mb. The chief advantage of the SMD is the ease with which 80 MB or more of information can be made available simply by replacing one disk pack on the drive with another.

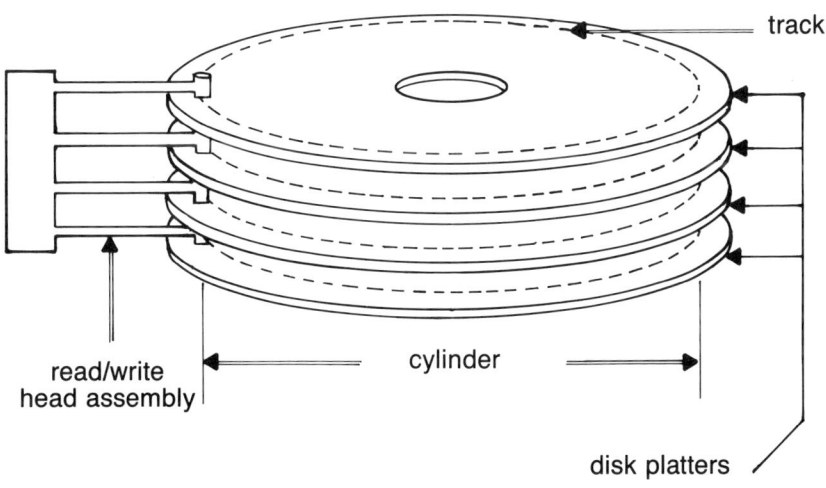

FIGURE 2-3 The read/write heads move together in the radial direction of the disk platter by the access arm. The stack of tracks (four in this drawing) traversed by the heads in one rotation of the disk forms a cylinder. Information is recorded in cylinders so that all heads are put to work in every read/write operation, thus increasing the data transfer rate.

Winchester Disks

SMD drives were the principal mass storage devices for minicomputers, such as nuclear medicine computers, through the mid-1980s. Today, Winchester disks have replaced the SMD as the mass storage device of choice. A technologic breakthrough, Winchester disks enable the head to position precisely on each track and to read or write a tiny uniform-sized spot on the disk surface. The dimensions of Winchester disks are much more compact than the SMD, but its storage capacity is several times greater than a conventional disk drive of comparable physical size. While 200 Mb is the practical limit for most SMD-type disk storage devices, the storage capacity of Winchester disks varies from a modest 20 Mb on the personal computers and up to 900 Mb in those used on the large computers.

Similar to disk platters in a SMD, a Winchester disk is made up of one or more aluminum platters coated with a magnetic recording medium. Unlike conventional disk drives, Winchester disk platters are permanently mounted on the disk drive and protected in a sealed housing. One of the reasons Winchester disks are able to achieve such a high storage capacity is because their read/write heads are placed even closer to the surface of the disk surface than the heads on the SMD drives. To avoid harmful contaminants from entering the disk chamber and scratching the head or the disk surface, the Winchester disks are assembled in a dust free room.

The advantages of the Winchester disk are its high storage capacity and fast access time. The main disadvantage of Winchester disk drives is that the disk platters are non-removable. In case of a disk drive failure, a large quantity of information is locked inside and most likely rendered useless during repair. Therefore, backup of information stored in Winchester disks cannot be overemphasized. As a guard against losing valuable data from machine malfunctions, many sophisticated Winchester disk drives contain a micro-processor and a small amount of memory which continuously monitors the performance of the drive and forewarns the user of any potential problems. Because of the increasing reliability and continual reduction in cost, the current generation of nuclear medicine computers have replaced SMDs with Winchester disks as the mass storage device.

Optimizing Hard Disk Performance

Many users may be surprised to learn that the disk storage system is a big determining factor on how responsive a computer can be. Common operations such as retrieving images from the disk to the display memory, loading programs from the disk onto the CPU memory to process the images, or saving the processed images on the disk take up a considerable portion of image processing time. The computer's sluggish response to the user requests is often due to delays in completing these input and output operations.

There are several ways to shorten the time spent waiting for the disk drive to perform its read/write duties. Of course, installing a fast Winchester disk on the computer helps to reduce the delays. However, we may still face the bottleneck imposed by the program and other hardware devices that govern how information is to be shuttled between the disk and the CPU memory. One hardware approach is utilizing a RAM disk as the staging buffer for frequently used programs and data to reduce the number of calls for disk services. Finally, regular reorganization of the layout of information on the disk (file defragmentation) can produce a startling increase in system performance.

File Defragmentation

When a new disk is put into service, various programs and image data, generically called files, are then neatly loaded onto the disk sequentially in contiguous blocks. When one or more files that are no longer needed are deleted, unslightly gaps are the results. When a new file is to be saved on the disk, the computer will pack as much data as it can into the first empty block it finds, it then puts the rest in the next free block, and so on. As a result, a single file broken into small pieces and scattered over many different locations (Fig. 2-4.) is said to be fragmented. File defragmentation refers to the process of re-grouping the location of the files on the disk so that parts belonging to the same file are consolidated into contiguous blocks. Just as straightening a disorganised desk makes it easier to find things, defragmentation of the files minimizes the head movement and yields faster file access.

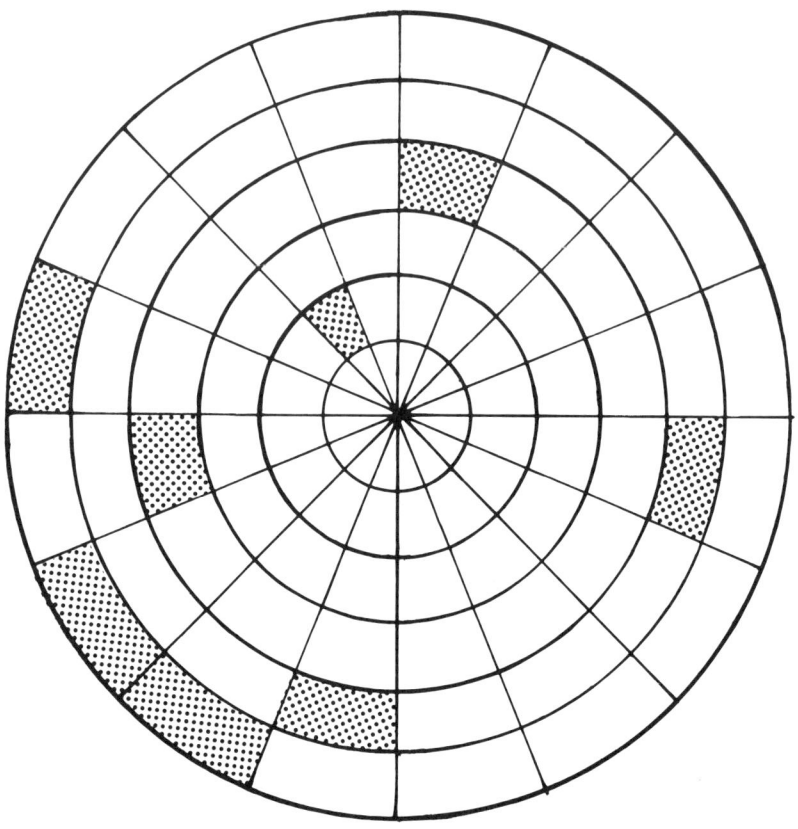

FIGURE 2-4 Frequent erasing and writing create non-contiguous blocks and cause parts of the same file to scatter over different tracks on the disk. A severely fragmented disk will slow down system response.

Although breaking a file into fragments helps to squeeze as much information as possible in every available space on a given disk, such a filing method imposes a penalty. Whenever you try to retrieve a file, the disk drive's read/write head has to scurry to pick up the pieces. The problem is especially severe for a high capacity disk that has been used for long periods with frequent addition and deletion of files; the time consumed by the read/write head to collect all the fragments can slow the system.

One way to perform file defragmentation is to transfer all the disk files to magnetic tapes, completely erase the disk of all files, and then copy the files on the magnetic tapes back to the disk. When copied back to the empty disk, parts belonging to the same file will be put in one contiguous location. Depending on the speed and capacity of the disk and magnetic tape drives, this method may require up to one day of user intervention to defragment a disk with several hundred megabytes of information.

There are commercially available programs, called disk optimizers, which will automatically collect fragments of each disk file to the CPU memory or to another storage media, erase the disk space they occupy, and rewrite the file back to the disk in the most efficient order. Once the disk optimizing program is initiated, all the disk files will be reorganized one after another without user intervention. Running one of these automatic file defragmentation programs overnight about once a month is one good way to minimize disk delays. One note of caution: any loss of power or interruption during disk optimization may cause loss of data or damage to the formatting structure.

RAM Disk

A RAM disk is a temporary storage system that uses a semiconductor RAM instead of a rotating disk platter as the storage media. Because reading and writing on the RAM disk happens purely by electronic means, involving no mechanical motions such as head movements and rotating platters, it provides a speed performance that cannot be matched by the fastest Winchester disk.

A RAM disk can be created by a piece of software which borrows some of the CPU memory to simulate the functions of a disk. This type of RAM disk is popular among personal computer users. However, one must be careful in reassigning the precious CPU memory for disk-emulation duties because memory assigned to a RAM disk is unavailable for executing programs. When the CPU memory is reduced, large programs often run inefficiently or not at all.

RAM disks usually found on an image processing computer use a separate set of MOS memory, independent of those in the CPU memory. The device used to control the read/write operations on the RAM disk also emulate many of the functions of a standard disk drive controller. Hence, programs written to work with a conventional disk drive can run on a computer with a RAM disk with little or no modifications.

The storage capacity of this type of RAM disk is large, varying from several hundred kilobytes to tens of megabytes. Unfortunately, information stored in the MOS memory of the RAM disk is not permanent; periodic saving of the processed data to the disk is necessary. However, users can see a dramatic gain in speed if they load all the needed programs and images onto the RAM disk before processing the images.

Floppy Disks

As the name suggests, *floppy disks* are flexible disk storage devices. The magnetic recording medium is coated on the surfaces of a mylar sheet, which gives it this flexible characteristic. The disk is enclosed inside a stiff envelope that has a lubricated interior felt lining to clean the disk surface as it rotates. In Figure 2-5, the jacket has

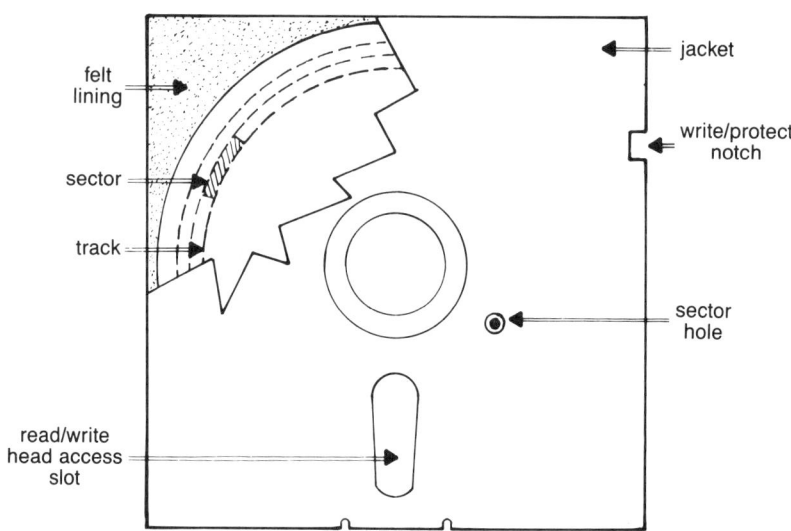

FIGURE 2-5 The anatomy of a 5-1/4-inch floppy disk.

a cut-out slot in the envelope, which exposes the disk to the access arm for read/write operations.

When inserted into the disk drive, the floppy disk is clamped onto the spindle. Due to the fluttering of the floppy disk during rotation, floppy disk drives rotate at only about 360 rpm, one-tenth the speed of hard disk drives. A slower rotation speed means that the read/write head takes more time to find an address on the disk, and more time for information to be written onto or read from the disk. A read or write operation for a 64 x 64 pixel 16-bit deep image takes several seconds or more to complete, while the same operation on a hard disk may take only 0.1 to 0.3 seconds. Unlike the read/write head on a hard disk, which skims above the disk surface with a cushion of air, the read/write head on the floppy disk actually comes in contact with the disk surface. As a result, they wear each other out. Typically the floppy disk wears out after several hours of actual read/write operations, while the magnetic head wears out after several hundred hours.

Floppy disks were first introduced with an 8-inch diameter. The standard single-density format of an 8-inch floppy disk holds 256 KB on a surface. The double-density format has the same number of tracks and sectors on a disk surface, but twice as many bytes are squeezed into each sector to give storage capacity of 512 KB on each surface. If the disk drive supports two read/write heads, one on each surface of the disk, the total storage capacity of a double-sided 8-inch floppy disk is 512 KB for the single-density format and 1 MB for the double-density format.

Another distinction of floppy disks is the manner in which the sector numbers are identified in each track. The now extinct hard-sectored floppy disks had a hole punched between each sector to help the access arm locate the sectors. The soft-sectored floppy disks have only one hole punched in the disk; sectors are laid out on each track by the software in a step called *formatting*, which must be done before a new disk can be used.

Floppy disks were originally designed as a temporary and convenient means for backup of small data sets and program instructions. The arrival of micro-computers has changed this original intent. Micro-computers use floppy disks with 5.25-inch diameters as their principal means of archiving data and programs. A 5.25-inch floppy disk, also known as a diskette, holds from about 140 KB to over 1 MB, depending on the recording density and whether one or both sides of the disk surface are used. An avid micro-computer user may keep several hundred diskettes of programs and data in his library.

The most recent type of floppy disk used in micro-computers measures about 3.50-inches in diameter. It has a hard plastic protective shell, instead of a flexible jacket, and a metal plate covers the head slot. These 3.50-inch floppy disks are called micro-floppy disks and can hold from 400 KB to 1 MB on each side to give a total storage capacity of up to 2 MB for a double-sided disk drive. There are micro-floppy disks in the developmental stage that can hold up to 6 MB. These rugged micro-floppy disks with ever increasing capacity are rapidly pushing the 5.25-inch diskettes into obsolescence as the 5.25-inch floppies did to the 8-inch floppies a few years ago.

THE FUTURE OF MAGNETIC

DISK TECHNOLOGY

Current magnetic disk technology is making incremental improvements by packing more data into smaller spaces. Because the magnetic field diverges from the magnetic recording head (Fig. 2-6) and cannot be focused, the only means to achieve higher recording density is to shrink the size of the head and to fly the head closer to the disk. Already, the relative speed and distance between the head and the disk platter is analogous to a jumbo jet flying at 500 miles per hour at 0.1 inch off the ground. Pushing the magnetic head much closer to the disk surface will require new technology to solve severe wear and tear problems at the head-disk interface. Meanwhile, an alternative magnetic recording method, perpendicular recording, has shown considerable promise to triple current recording density.

Perpendicular Recording

To date, magnetic recording has been done with magnetic fields, or bits, oriented in the same plane as the disk platter. Because the fields lie end-to-end, they tend to neutralize one another, particu-

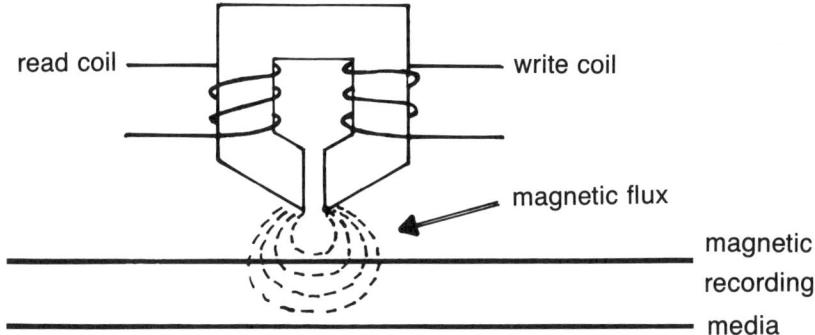

FIGURE 2-6 The magnetic flux diverges from the read/write head. In order to produce high-recording density, the read/write head must fly close to the disk surface to make small magnetized spots. In the past decade, flying heights plunged from 800 to 6 microinches.

larly when like poles are adjacent to one another. This self-demagnetization effect thus limits the recording density. Perpendicular recording orients the magnetic fields at right angles to the plane of the disk (Fig. 2-7). With perpendicular recording, self-demagnetization is much less of a problem because the adjacent mag-

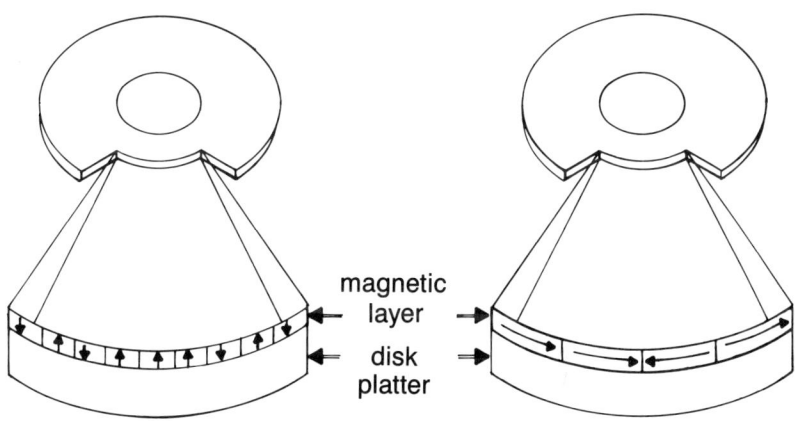

FIGURE 2-7 The new vertical recording technique can pack more data on a disk by placing magnetic domains perpendicular to the surface instead of horizontally as is currently done.

netic fields do not oppose each other. In addition, the magnetic coatings on the disk platters for perpendicular recording can be made much thicker and thus should be easier to produce with fewer defects. Unfortunately, progress in perfecting the perpendicular recording technique has been rather slow. One reason is the difficulty in constructing a mechanical system that moves the magnetic recording head to positions accurately, repeatedly, and rapidly for reading and writing at high densities. At the time of this writing, commercial models are just becoming available.

OPTICAL DISKS

Optical disks, the latest computer mass storage devices, are still in their infancy. However, the first few commercially available optical disk drives already offer several times the storage capacity of today's highest capacity Winchester drives. For example, a 5.25-inch diameter optical disk, costing approximately $150, can store 1 gigabytes (1 billion bytes) of data on each side of the platter, equivalent to 200,000 frames of 64 x 64 16-bit images. An optical disk "juke box", holding 10 or more of these platters, can store over 2 million images with an image retrieval time of less than 10 seconds.

Optical disks are formatted during the manufacturing process by a stamping machine, which impresses thousands of grooves on the disk surface. A 5.25-inch diameter optical disk may have 40,000 or more tracks stamped on one surface. At this early stage of development, various manufacturers are using widely different techniques to record information onto optical disks. However, all of these recording techniques take advantage of the high intensity and narrow diameter of laser beams. One of the techniques used to enter data onto a non-erasable optical disk is illustrated in Figure 2-8. To write data onto the disk, a beam of high intensity laser is focused on a spot of approximately 1 micron in diameter. Intense heat from the laser softens the metal layer and decomposes the polymer in its path into gaseous products. The gas pressure builds up due to the highly localized heating, and pushes up on the softened metal layer, which creates a bubble. To read the recorded information, the laser in low-intensity mode is focused onto the disk. The presence of a bubble reduces the intensity of the beam reflected

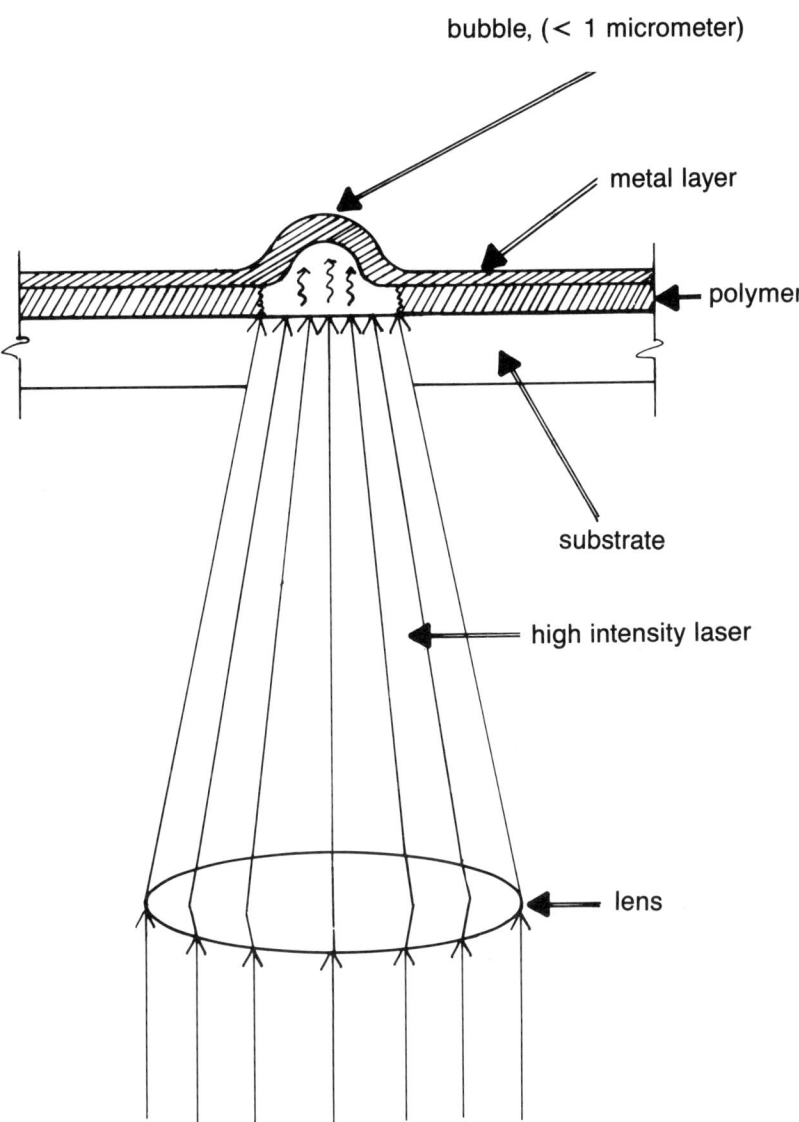

FIGURE 2-8 Intense heating by the laser softens the metal layer and vaporizes the polymer. The vapor pressure pushes up the metal layer and forms a bubble.

toward the read/write head. We can arbitrarily call a spot with a reduced reflection intensity a bit with a value of 1, and the spot with no change in the reflection intensity a bit with a value of 0. The disk surface can be written on only once because the bubbles will remain permanently on the disk surface. The generic name for the non-erasable optical disk is the WORM (Write Once Read Many) disk. WORM disks are ideal for archival purposes because information once recorded on the disk becomes permanent and will not be subjected to accidental erasures.

A technique that combines perpendicular magnetic recording with the laser technology to produce an erasable read/write optical disk is illustrated in Figure 2-9. The magnetic-optic layer is composed of a special blend of rare-earth transition metals, whose magnetic polarity can be easily rotated in an elevated temperature. To record data onto the disk, a steady magnetic field is applied perpendicularly to the disk. When a high-intensity laser beam is focused on a spot in a recording track, the intense heat brought on by the laser enables the externally applied magnetic field to invert the magnetic polarity of the metals within that laser heated spot.

To read the recorded information, a beam of low-intensity polarized laser is focused on the spots. The spots (i.e., the bits) with unchanged magnetic polarity rotate the polarized laser to one direction, while those spots with inverted magnetic polarity rotate the polarized laser to a different direction. The direction of the rotated light thus represents binary zeroes and ones. The previously recorded information can be erased simply by applying a strong external magnetic field to the disk and forcing the magnetic polarity of all spots to orient in one direction.

In spite of the enormous storage capacity, optical disk technology is still far from solving our data storage problems. The data access time is longer than that of the Winchester disks. The WORM disks are suitable for storing large quantities of data that need to be kept over a long period of time, but that do not require high speed access. An example of such an application is a patient file retrieval system requiring long term storage and an access time of several seconds. Non-erasable optical disks have only limited use as auxiliary storage because data or program instructions cannot be continually updated.

MASS STORAGE DEVICES

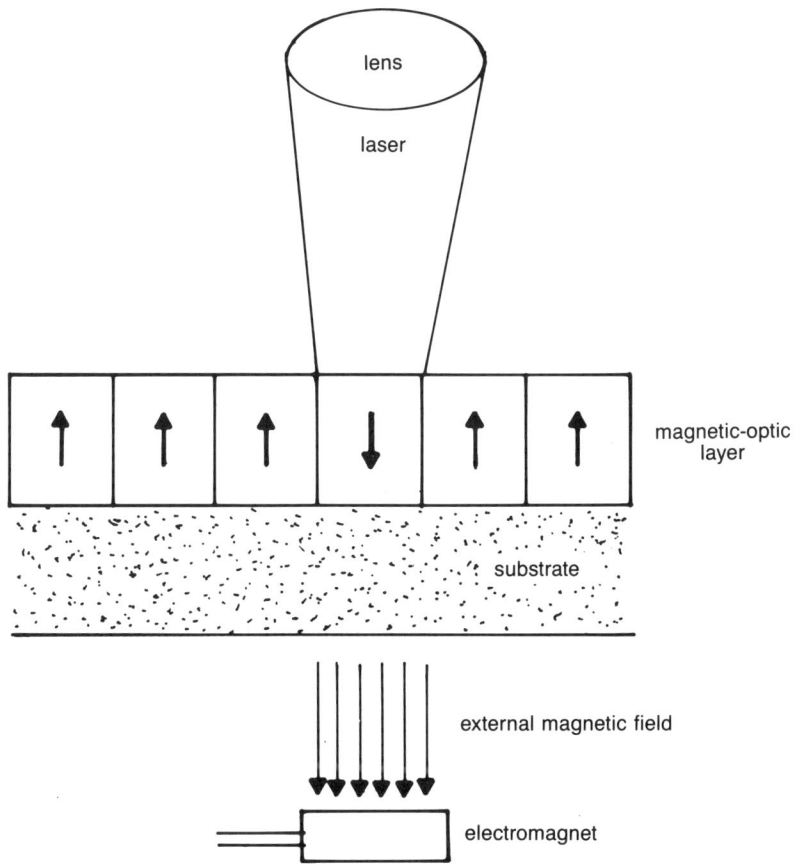

FIGURE 2-9 An erasable optical disk contains a magnetic-optic layer. Upon heating by the laser, the magnetic polarity can be flipped to the opposite direction by an external magnetic field.

MAGNETIC TAPE DRIVES

Magnetic tape drives are synonymous with the sequential access storage device. Although magnetic tapes are commonly perceived as a mass storage media for archival of data not requiring immediate access, they are also utilized as a convenient means for information exchange between computers because the tape format has been standardized over the last 30 years, and as a backup device to information stored on the magnetic disk.

The variety of magnetic tape systems available today can be classified according to the width of the tape and the tape-mounting mechanism on the drive. The 0.50-inch *reel-to-reel* magnetic tape drives have been the backbone of mass storage devices since the early 1950s due to their high storage capacity. The *cartridge* tape drives with either a 0.25-inch or a 0.50-inch wide tape housed inside a plastic cartridge assembly are now challenging the reel-to-reel tape drives as the mass storage device of choice because of its compactness, high storage capacity and convenience. The 0.15-inch *audiocassette* tape drives were once tried as storage devices on personal computers. Due to their small storage capacity, low speed, and poor reliability, they never enjoyed much popularity even among the most budget-minded home computer users.

Reel-to-Reel Tape Drives

In spite of the number of types of tape devices, the recording and playback techniques are basically the same. The operating principles of magnetic tape drives are described using the reel-to-reel drive as an example because they are the most widely used variety. Figure 2-10 shows that a magnetic tape consists of a magnetic coating on one side of a mylar tape (0.50 inch wide and up to 3600 feet long) in a 10-inch diameter reel. A piece of silver reflective tape is adhered to the beginning and near the end of the tape to alert a light sensor to prevent the tape transport mechanism from over-running. The amount of information that can be stored on a reel of tape is determined by the number of recording tracks on the surface of the tape, the recording density on each track, and the length of the tracks, i.e., the length of the tape.

The standard format divides the width of the tape into nine tracks, parallel to the length of the tape. There is one read/write head provided for each recording track. An electric current passes through the read/write head and produces a magnetic field which in turn produces a magnetized spot in the track directly in front of the head. Reversing the direction of electric current through the read/write head demagnetizes a spot on the tape. After each write operation, the previously recorded information is replaced by a new row of nine spots (bits) which is either magnetized or demagnetized to represent binary zeroes or ones. The number of rows of magne-

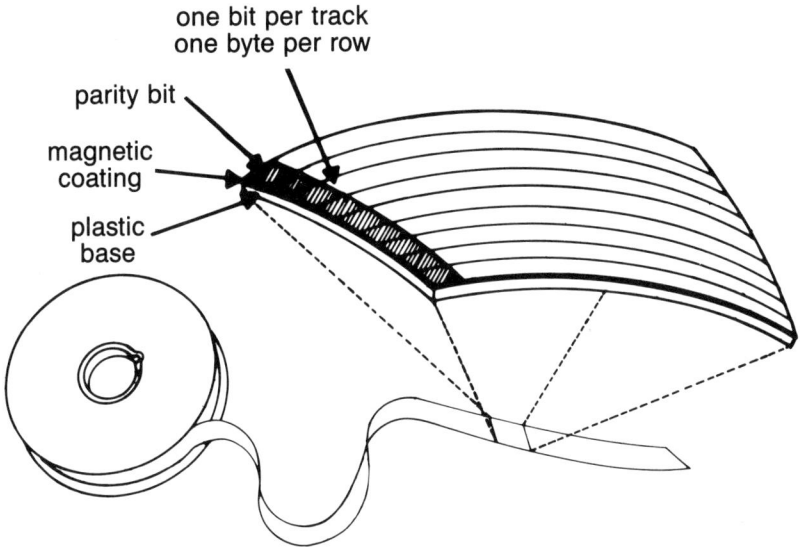

FIGURE 2-10 The surface of a conventional tape is divided into nine tracks along its length. A row of magnetized spots across eight of the tracks form 1 byte of information. The ninth spot, called the parity bit, is used for error checking.

tized spots per unit length of tape is called the linear density and is expressed in bits per inch (bpi). Common linear densities currently is use are 1600 and 6250 bpi. The standard varieties on minicomputers such as those in nuclear medicine departments are nine-track 1600 bpi tape drives. On these nine-track tape drives, eight tracks across the width of the tape are written simultaneously to record 1 byte of data, and the ninth track is used for error checking. With the tape drive operating at 1600 bpi, it is recording 1600 bytes of data onto each inch of the tape. Hence, up to 45 MB of data can be stored in a reel with 2400 feet of tape. Actually the effective stroage capacity is about 40 MB because gaps and other markings are placed on the tape to separate adjacent sets of data.

To increase the recording density of magnetic tapes, both the linear density and the number of tracks must be increased. Reel-to-reel tape drives featuring 34 tracks and 20,000 bpi have been made. Unfortunately, commercial production of such high-density reel-to-reel tape drive mechanisms have been hampered by reliability problems. A major roadblock to widespread use of high-density reel-to-reel tape drives is the inadequacy of the tape transport mechanisms to align the tape precisely in front of the read/write heads. The relatively low-density tape drives today have a large tolerance for misalignment of a track from its corresponding read/write head. For a tape drive to read or write 20,000 bpi on each of 34 tracks across a 0.50-inch wide tape, the guiding and head positioning mechanism requires great precision because there is not much room for error between two tracks.

Data recording on a magnetic tape is more susceptible to errors than data recording on disk. One of the techniques used to detect errors on magnetic tape is the parity check. The computer program used to instruct the tape drive to write data on the magnetic tape can impose a condition that a row must have an odd or even number of bits set to 1. The constraint that only an odd number of 1-bits is permitted in any one row is called the odd parity, while the even parity requires that there must be an even number of 1-bits across a row. Suppose, we have an odd parity constraint on a data recording. One of the tracks in the tape is reserved to hold a parity bit, which is set to 1, if the number of 1-bits across the row is even, and set to a 0 if a row already has an odd number of 1-bits. During the read operation, the data are considered valid only if there is an odd number of 1-bits across a row, and the computer will give a parity error message if an even number of 1-bits is detected.

Another technique to ensure correct taping of data is *redundant recording*, whereby each set of data is consecutively recorded on tape twice. If an error was found in one of the two sets of data during the read operation, then the computer would transfer the set with no errors to the memory and ignore the other set. The read operation is successful only if one of the two sets of data is free from error. The computer will halt if both sets of data contain errors.

There are several ways to minimize errors on magnetic tape:

1. Avoid touching the recording surface of the magnetic tape with your hands, as your finger smudge will interfere with correct reading and writing by the magnetic heads on the tape drive.
2. Clean the magnetic read/write heads periodically with

alcohol and a cotton swab to minimize the accumulation of dirt and dust on the surface.
3. If the magnetic tape is not going to be used for an extended period of time, e.g., 1 hour, it should be rewound and released of its tension. The section of tape in tension for a long period of time could be stretched more than the other sections. An unevenly stretched tape is one of the conditions that often leads to read errors.
4. Use tape with the linear density rated at least as high as the tape drive. If a tape is recording at 6,250 bpi, one should not use a tape rated for a lower density, e.g., 1,600 bpi.

Tape Cartridges

Tape cartridge drives are beginning to overtake the conventional reel-to-reel tape drives as the bulk storage device of choice. Tape cartridges contain either a 0.25-inch or a 0.50-inch wide tape wound in two spools inside a sealed plastic case. Cartridge tapes are mounted by simply inserting the entire cartridge into a slot, and there is no manual threading of tape through the read/write head assembly, as is the case for reel-to-reel magnetic tape units. They are more compact and better protected against dirt. Furthermore, many of the 0.50-inch cartridge tape drives are out-performing the reel-to-reel tape in their storage capacity. A cartridge is about the size of the hand; it contains about 600 feet of 0.50-inch wide magnetic tape wound around two spools inside. There may be 24 tracks across the width and up to 12,000 bpi along the length of the tape, giving the cartridge capacity from 90 MB to 300 MB. As a comparison, the capacity of a reel of 2400 feet magnetic tape recording at 1600 bpi is about 40 MB. The 0.25-inch wide cartridge tapes have a lower recording density, but the storage capacity is still in the 20 to 60 MB range, comparable to the reel-to-reel tape capacity. However, the read/write operations on the cartridge tapes are much slower than their reel-to-reel tapes, and there are no standardized formats for data recording at the present time. Hence, using the cartridge tape as a media for information interchange is possible only among users with computers made by the same manufacturer at the present time.

CONCLUSION

With the different mass storage devices discussed above, I speculate that optical disks will become the dominant bulk-storage device by the mid 1990s, while magnetic tapes will serve as backup to optical disks. This speculation is not too far-fetched when we consider that one optical disk holds as much information as 50 reels of 0.50-inch 1600 bpi tape, and a juke box containing 10 optical disks holds the equivalent of 500 reels of tape. All it takes is about 10 seconds to retrieve information from the juke box. If the information stored on magnetic tapes, the operator would have to search for the proper tape reel in a small warehouse, come back to mount the tape, and then sequentially read the data into memory. This process could take more than 20 minutes. Besides faster retrieval and less operator intervention, large volumes of data can be kept in a small building facility by compacting them into optical disks.

Unless the erasable optical disk technology undergoes some radical improvements, Winchester disks will continue to serve as the principle mass storage devices into the early 1990s, while high-density cartridge tapes will find wider use as a reliable and cost-effective alternative to reel-to-reel magnetic tapes for bulk storage. Three and one-half inch floppy disks will become the standard temporary storage media.

CHAPTER

3

INPUT AND OUTPUT DEVICES

INTRODUCTION

Input devices are peripheral equipment, which enable the operator to enter instructions and data into the computer. Common input devices in a nuclear medicine computer include keyboard terminals, analog-to-digital converters (AC/DCs), light pens, mice, trackballs, and joysticks. *Output devices* are electronic gadgets used by the computer to display the results. Keyboard terminals, video monitors, and printers are familiar output devices to nuclear medicine computer users. Many devices, such as keyboard terminals and modems, serve a dual role as both the input channel for entering data and instructions to the computer, and as an output channel for the results. For this reason, the class of devices used for communicating information between the computer and the outside world is collectively called the input/output (I/O) devices. Some people consider magnetic disks and tapes to be I/O devices as well, because these devices are used to hold output from the CPU, as well as feed program instructions and data for processing. As the usage of peripheral devices becomes increasingly specialized, magnetic disks and tapes will be regarded more as peripheral mass storage devices than as I/O devices.

INPUT DEVICES

Keyboard Terminals

The keyboard terminal is a control console for the user to enter programs, data, or commands to the computer. The most common type of keyboard terminal is the video display terminal (VDT); it consists of a video display monitor and a typewriter-like keyboard. In addition to the usual typewriter keys, some terminals have a numeric keypad, much like the nine-key adding machine, and a number of special-function keys. These special-function keys can be programmed to initiate a chain of commands one after another to the computer and thus saves the operator much repetitive typing, since only one key needs to be struck.

Whenever a key is struck by the user, a binary code unique to that key is generated. This binary code, when interpreted by a special ROM called a character generator, produces on the video screen a dot pattern mimicking a letter, a numeral or a graphics symbol. The video display screen typically measures 12 inches diagonally, and displays 25 lines of 80 characters each. The current video monitors offer character displays in a green or amber color against a black background, instead of the traditional black and white display. Since the light emitted by the phosphor on the video screen fades away after a fraction of a second, the entire screen display must be refreshed at least 30 or more times a second in order to minimize the amount of flickering. Nearly all stand-alone terminals have a small amount of memory, which allows the terminal electronics to refresh the video display and relieve the CPU from continually rewriting data on the screen. By increasing the memory size and adding a microprocessor to the terminal, we obtain an intelligent terminal which allows the user to edit text and perform a limited amount of arithmetic.

The speed with which a terminal sends data out or accepts data from the computer is specified by its *baud rate*. The baud rate can be simply defined as the number of bits per second transmitted through the cable between the computer and the terminal. In the rigorous definition of the baud rate, one baud does not always equal 1 bit per second. Instead of laboring on the exact definition of a baud, here are three intuitive examples. Most of the prevalent terminals communicate with the computer at 9600 baud. However, the older terminals and those communicate with the computer via a modem have communication speeds varying from 300 to 2400 baud. At 300 baud, you need to wait patiently for each character to pop up on the screen. At 2400 baud, your eyes can keep up with the printing of one line after another. However, at 9600 baud, a screen full of characters can roll up in about one second.

INPUT AND OUTPUT DEVICES   45

Modems And Acoustic Couplers

If a terminal is located too far away from the computer for direct cable connection, telephone cables are utilized as the communication link. However, telephone lines are designed for the communication of analog electrical signals. Binary signals from the computer terminal will become badly distorted if they are sent through the telephone line. In order to take advantage of the extensive telephone cable system as the communication pathway, the terminal requires either a *modem*, or, in the grand old days, an *acoustic coupler* to convert its output digital data into electrical pulses for transmission over the telephone lines to the computer. Conversely, either a modem or an acoustic coupler is needed to convert electrical pulses sent through the telephone lines from the computer into digital data, before forwarding them to the terminal.

Acoustic Couplers

Acoustic couplers are all but extinct in modern computer communication devices, but it is instructive to review its operational principles to better understand how the computer communicates with the outside world. To use an acoustic coupler as a communication linkage with the computer, the telephone handset is placed snugly in the rubber receptacles of the acoustic coupler. When a key in the terminal keyboard is pressed down, the binary output signal is converted by the acoustic coupler into one of two audio tones (two different sound frequencies), one frequency for binary ones and a different frequency for binary zeroes. When the tone is picked up by the telephone handset, the diaphragm inside the handset converts the tone to an electrical signal for transmission over the telephone lines. Of course, the frequency of the electrical signal corresponding to the tone produced by 1 bit is different from the frequency of the electrical signal produced by 0 bit. Upon reaching the receiving station at the destination computer, the original bit pattern is reassembled by converting the incoming electrical signals to ones and zeroes according to their frequencies. The advantage of acoustic couplers is their simplicity and low cost. However, signals transmitted via an acoustic coupler are more subject to noise and a higher rate of errors. The transmission speed is also slow, limited to 300 baud.

Modems

Modems are more sophisticated than acoustic couplers. They communicate with the computer at a much higher speed, make fewer errors, and are less susceptible to noise. The name modem is a contraction for modulation and demodulation. Unlike acoustic couplers, which require a telephone handset as an intermediary to convert digital data into analog electrical signals, modems use their own electronic circuitry to convert the binary signals directly into electrical signals for transmission. A modem produces a single continuous electrical wave called a *carrier* wave or frequency for transmission. This carrier wave is then re-shaped by the digital modulator so that each signal variation is interpreted by the receiver to be either 0 or 1. Modulation is a fancy term for a process that changes the amplitude, phase, or frequency of one sinusoidal wave in accordance with another wave. Digital modulation is the process by which the analog carrier wave produced by the modem is modified according to the bit pattern of the digital output signals from the terminal.

The three basic techniques to modulate the carrier wave — amplitude modulation (AM), frequency modulation (FM), and phase modulation (PM) — are illustrated in Figure 3-1. In AM modulation, the signal strength or height of the carrier wave is changed between high and low depending on the value of the bit received, high amplitude for a 1-bit and low amplitude for a 0-bit, for example. Amplitude modulation is simple but rarely used in modems because this technique is only suitable for low-speed transmission and is vulnerable to noise interference.

Phase modulation has good noise tolerance and is used for transmission at 9600 baud and above. The PM process changes the phase angle but keeps the amplitude and frequency of the carrier wave intact. High speed transmission with the PM technique is possible because each phase shift can be used to represent two or more bits. For example, phase shifts of 90, 180, 270, or 360 degrees can be used to represent two bits having values of 00, 01, 10, and 11, respectively. The disadvantage of PM is the need for complex encoding and decoding circuitry. Frequency modulation, sometimes known as the frequency-shift-keying (FSK) technique, works by shifting the carrier frequency above or below a reference frequency while keeping the amplitude and phase constant. The FSK technique is wide-

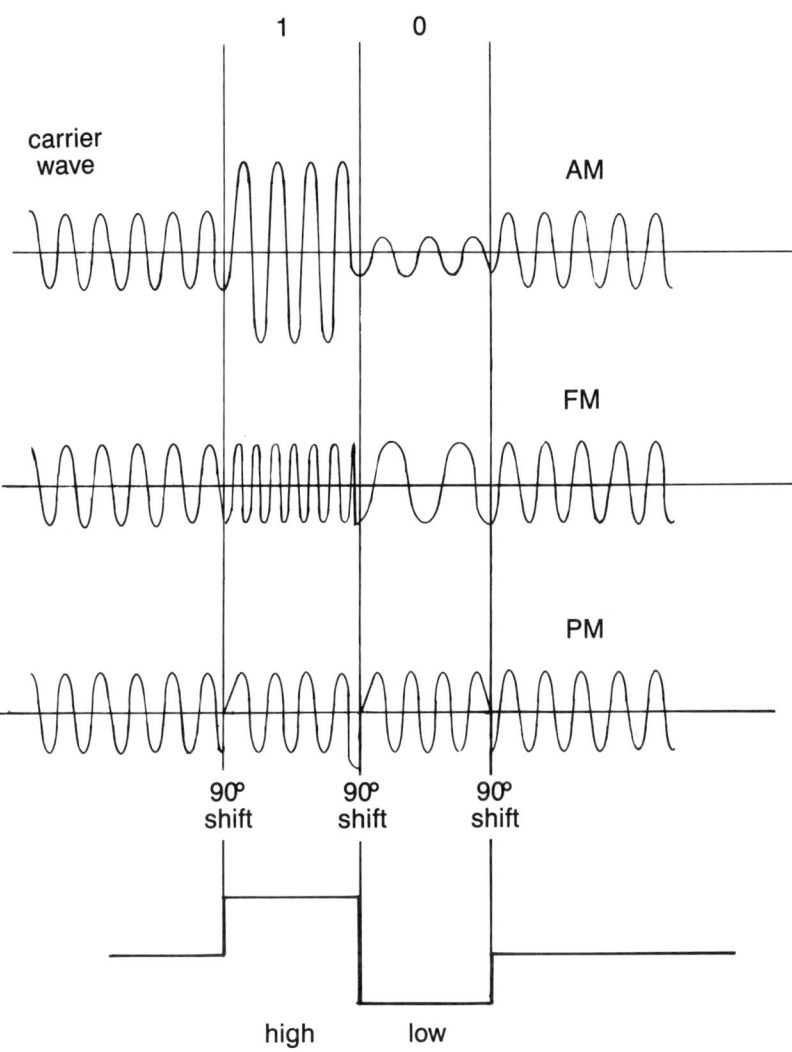

FIGURE 3-1 Of the three methods of modulating carrier wave in a modem, amplitude modulation is no longer used. Frequency modulation is the predominant methods for the 1200 and 2400 baud modems, while phase modulation is used in modems operating at 9600 baud and higher.

ly used with modems for data transmission at 1200 to 2400 baud due to its relatively simple design and modest cost.

Two more descriptive characteristics of modems should be noted. Information coded by the modem can be transmitted by one of two timing methods—asynchronous and synchronous. Using the asynchronous method of transmission, bits of data are sent out in bursts at random time intervals. The receiver is alerted to the beginning and ending of each burst of data by a start and a stop signal. The asynchronous transmission rates over telephone lines are typically between 1200 to 2400 baud, although modems with 9600 baud are becoming common. Synchronous transmission moves data according to a clocking signal in a highly ordered sequence. Encoding and decoding are precisely coordinated with the beginning and ending timing marks. Synchronous transmission requires sophisticated software and special communication hardware. The normal speech telephone lines are not adequate for communication rates above 9600 baud. For these reasons, special telephone lines are required for high speed synchronous transmissions.

Both the asynchronous and synchronous transmission methods can operate in either half-duplex or full-duplex modes. Half-duplex permits transmission in one direction at a time. If the terminal is sending, the computer can only receive and not transmit. Conversely, while the computer is sending data to the terminal, the terminal is prohibited from transmitting until the computer is done. Under full-duplex, both the computer and terminal can transmit and receive at the same time.

Analog-To-Digital Converters

In a nuclear medicine computer system, counts from a radionuclide study are taken from the output of a gamma camera to the computer for processing. However, the signals representing the position and energy information of each count from a gamma camera are analog electrical voltage pulses. In order for the numerical value of an analog voltage pulse to be read into the computer, it must first be converted into a binary code that is recognizable to the computer. The process of changing an analog signal to a digital representation is called *analog-to-digital* conversion (ADC). The ADC is an interface device between the gamma camera and the computer that converts an analog electric signal from the gamma camera to a binary code that is recognized by the computer.

To distinguish the difference between an analog signal and a digital signal, an analog signal, such as a voltage pulse from the gamma camera, can be represented by a continuous curve whose magnitude varies continuously throughout the duration of the signal as shown in Figure 3-2. A digital signal, on the other hand, has only one of two possible discrete values throughout the duration of the signal. The term *discrete* means that the time it takes for the signal to make a transition from the low state to the high state is negligibly small compared to the duration of the signal. In analog-to-digital

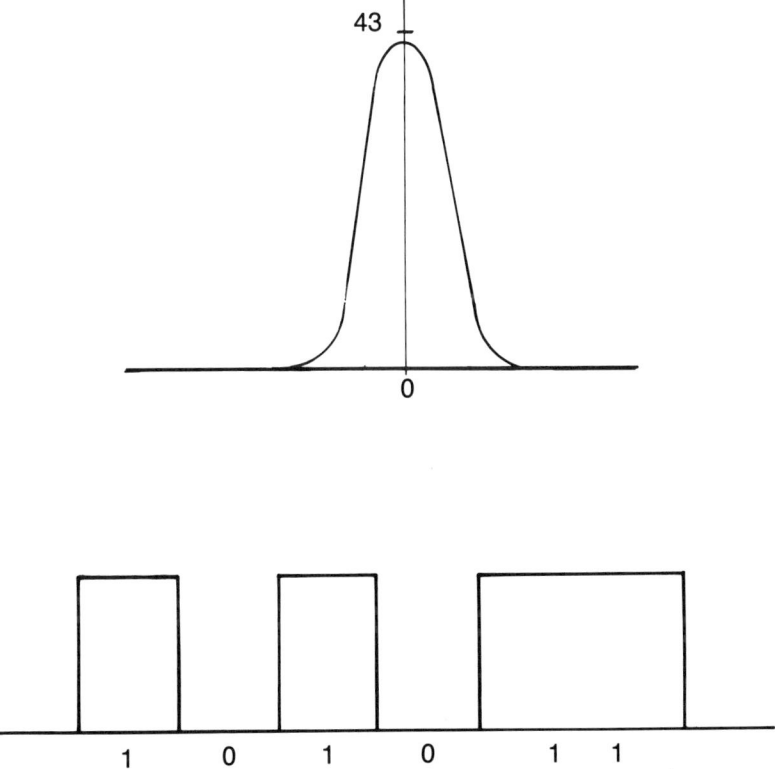

FIGURE 3-2 The binary signal 101011 is the digital equivalent of the analog signal 43.

conversion, an analog signal is changed to a train of digital pulses whose binary sum equals the magnitude of the analog signal.

There is a number of different ADC converters. The ADC connected to a joystick is the slower variety, which explains why the motion of many joystick-controlled displays on the screen frequently lag behind the hand motion. The ADC interfaced to a gamma camera is the high-speed successive approximation type capable of converting over 100,000 analog signals per second. Successive approximation of ADC work is discussed further in Appendix B.

OUTPUT DEVICES

Screen Pointing Devices

Every image processing computer has one or more input devices to supplement the keyboard for screen pointing and drawing functions. Lightpens, mice, trackballs, and joysticks are all screen pointing devices used in nuclear medicine computers. These devices were designed to ease human control of the cursor movements on the video monitor. Their operational principles and degrees of success in achieving the design goal are discussed briefly as follows.

Light Pens

Readers unfamiliar with the operational principles of video display should read the section on image display monitors before reading this section on light pens.

The light pen works with the video display controller and the electron beam that sweeps across the monitor screen as shown in Figure 3-3. The coordinates of the location pointed at by the pen are determined by the time that the electron beam took to move from the upper left hand corner of the video screen to the position in front of the pen. Thus, the light pen can be thought of as a stop watch with a light sensitive on/off switch. When the electron beam is at the starting position, the clock is set to zero and then allowed to run as the beam sweeps from left to right down the screen. When the beam strikes the phosphors in front of the light pen, a flash of light causes a photodetector inside the pen to emit an electric pulse, which then triggers a stop signal to the clock, and the elapsed time is noted. Because the scanning speed is known, we can calculate the length

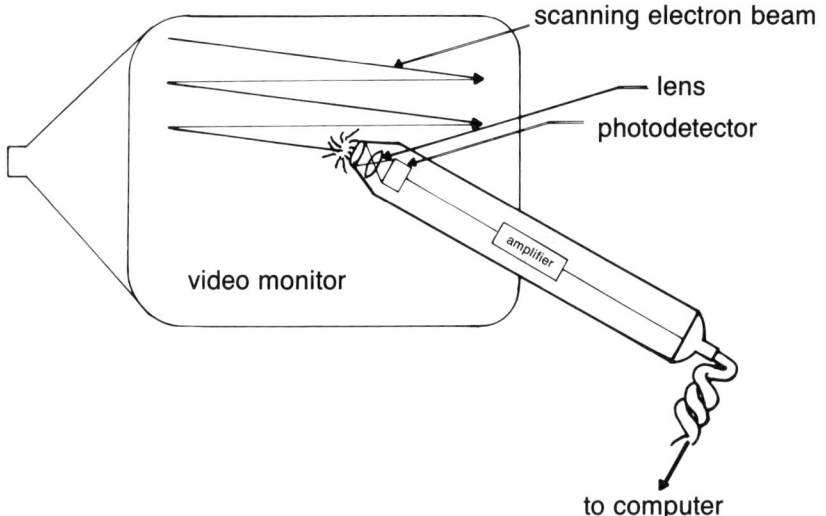

FIGURE 3-3 The light pen works like a stop watch. It measures the time for the electron beam to travel from the upper left corner of the screen to the position of the light pen. Location of the light pen is then calculated using the elapsed time, scan speed, and scan pattern of the electron beam.

of the track swept by the electron beam in that time interval. Because we also know the precise route of travel, the location of the flash can be easily determined.

The light pen might seem as natural as a ballpoint pen for pointing and drawing. Due to its ergonomic drawbacks, however, light pens are not used on the current nuclear medicine computers. First, the pens make the user work against gravity with the arm stretched out, and the user has to constantly battle the coiled cord to keep the pen from being tipped up towards the sky. In addition, the gap between the lens of the pen and the phosphors behind the monitor's glass screen make it difficult to aim the pen at the desired locations. Nevertheless, we may see light pens reincarnated in computerized nuclear medicine departments as bar code readers to identify codes on radiopharmaceutical labels and on patient hospital charts. (Bar code readers emit light and measure the reflections from the labels.)

Mice, Trackballs, and Joysticks

The construction and operational principles of mice, trackballs, and joysticks are very similar. They differ mostly in the hand motions required to control these devices. Figure 3-4 shows how a mechanical mouse works. There are two rollers placed perpendicularly to each other and pressed against the surface of a ball. Attached to the end of each roller is a disk with electrical contact points along the rim. As the mouse is moved about on the desk, the ball rotates and turns the disks. When the disks rotate, different contact points touch the contact bars on the housing, and produce a range of voltage signals. The signals are then calibrated to coordinate with the locations of the cursor on the screen.

The mouse is probably the most versatile screen pointing and drawing device. With practice, the cursor can be steered by a mouse to draw a complicated pattern on the screen. If you do not have enough desk space for a mouse to move around, turn the mouse on its back, rub the ball around in its stationary housing, and you obtain a trackball. A trackball offers the same precise control of cursor movements as the mouse, except that it does not require extra desk space to move around on. If your hand becomes sore from rubbing the trackball, attach a rod on top of the trackball for steering, and you obtain a joystick. Joysticks are slightly more difficult to use and less precise than trackballs and mice because the steering rod limits

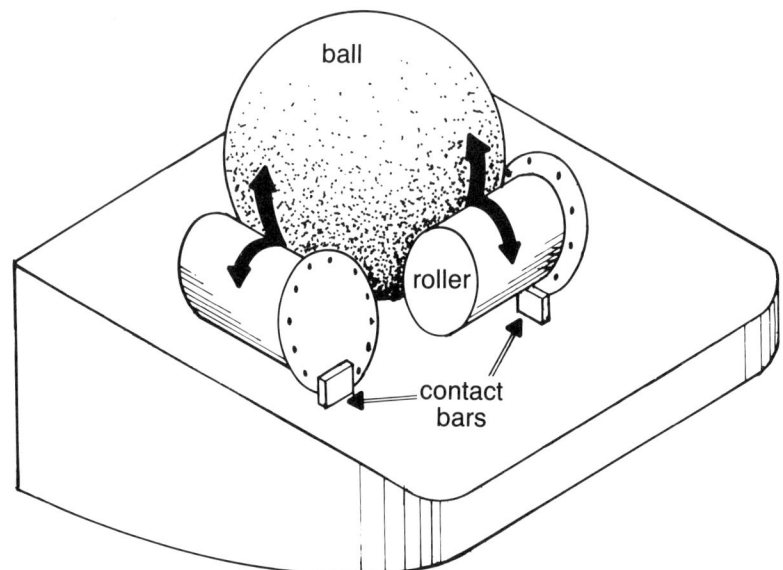

FIGURE 3-4 The essential elements of a mechanical mouse.

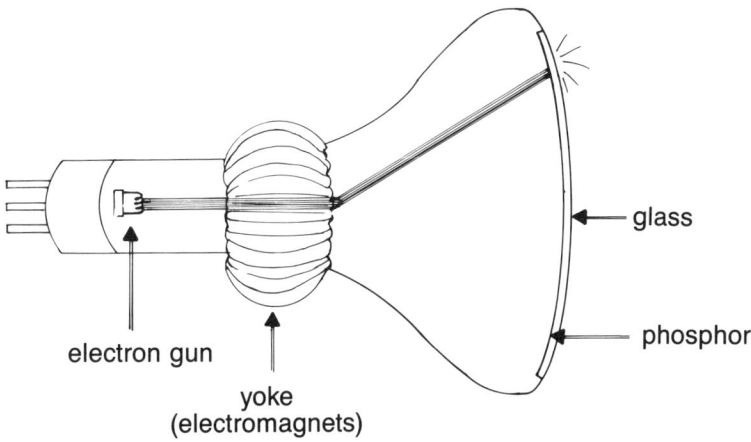

FIGURE 3-5 The principal components of a monochrome monitor. The beam of electrons emitted from the electron gun is steered by the yoke (pairs of electromagnets) to strike the phosphors on the viewing screen to produce a luminous image.

the rotation of the ball to less than 180° in both directions. Also, two hands are required to operate the joystick, one hand for steering and the other hand for pushing a button or a key to accept the cursor position. With a trackball or a mouse, the palm moves the ball, leaving the fingers free to click a button on its housing.

Image Display Monitors

High quality monitors are of paramount importance in a nuclear medicine computer system because the radionuclide images on the display monitor often form the basis for clinical diagnosis. While all monitors utilize the cathode ray tube (CRT) and raster scan technology, they vary widely in resolution and other performance features. A review of the complex raster scan process to produce video images will help in realizing the inherent limitations of CRT-displayed images.

Monochrome Display Monitors

A monochrome CRT, as illustrated in Figure 3-5, consists of three major components. The front end of the CRT is a glass screen coated with a layer of phosphors, which glow for about one-tenth of a second when struck by a beam of energetic electrons. If all the phosphors emit the same color of light, such as white, green, or amber, the display monitor is called monochrome. The electrons are emitted from an electron gun (located in the rear), which is maintained at several hundred volts negative to the phosphor screen. In some high resolution color monitors, the accelerating voltage can be as high as a thousand volts. When a stream of electrons is released from the electron gun and accelerated toward the phosphor screen, its direction of travel is controlled by the yoke which steers it to converge to a point on the screen. The landing spot of the electron beam on the screen is called a raster.

The yoke makes use of several pairs of electro-magnetic coils, which steer the electron beam in the horizontal and vertical directions (Fig. 3-6). At the start, the beam is directed to the upper left corner and is swept across the screen with a slight downward slope toward the right edge. When the beam reaches the right edge, it reverses the direction and quickly returns to the left edge. Once the beam is returned to the left edge of the screen, it repeats the sweep to the right edge, again at a downward angle. This trace pattern is repeated until the beam reaches the lower right corner of the screen. Then it returns quickly back to its starting point at the upper left corner and begins the down sweep cycle again. The standard video monitors use 525 such horizontal lines to form one frame of image on a full screen, while the high resolution monitors use 1024 lines. Very high resolution monitors utilizing 2048 lines are becoming available for the display of x-ray images.

Because light emitted from the phosphors fades away in such a small fraction of a second, the electron beam must refresh the screen very rapidly in order to reduce flickering of the image. The number of times per second that the electron beam makes a complete scan of the entire screen is called the *screen refresh rate* or the *frame rate*. For the display of high resolution images, the screen needs to have a refresh rate of at least 60 frames per second or 60 Hz in order to keep image flickers to an acceptable level. As a comparison, standard video monitors, such as home televisions, have a refresh rate of 30 Hz that is adequate for all soap opera viewing. Many monitors, notably commercial televisions, use a technique called *interlace*, which reduces the amount of screen flickers by breaking the horizontal scan into two parts, or fields. In the first part, the beam sweeps across the odd-numbered scan lines only, and on retrace scans the even-numbered lines. Thus, a frame consists of two fields produced by two scanning cycles. With interlace, the screen appears to refresh at twice the actual frame rate because our eyes cannot tell that only alternate lines are refreshed at each trace and retrace.

An image appears on the CRT because each raster on the screen emits light at different brightness levels when struck by the electron beam. The brightness of each raster depends on the intensity of the electron beam striking the phosphors, which in turn depends on the voltage applied to the electron gun—the higher the electron gun voltage, the higher the intensity of the electron beam, and the brighter each raster. A raster can be made completely black if the voltage applied to the electron gun is reduced to a minimum, and completely white if the electron gun shoots the phosphor screen at full blast. A continuous shade of gray from completely black to completely white can be produced by simply varying the electron beam intensity between the minimum and maximum. An image, which is actually

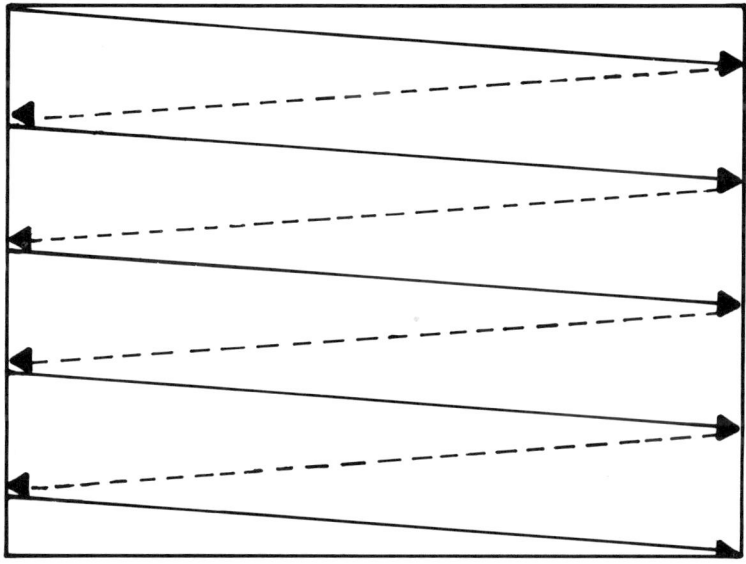

FIGURE 3-6 In a video monitor, the electron beam sweeps across the screen starting position and repeats the scan.

a mosaic made up of rasters of different shades of gray, results from the computer instructing a device called the video display controller to vary the voltage applied to the electron gun systematically. The display controller, acting according to instructions given by the computer, is synchronized with the horizontal and vertical sweeps of the electron beam so that the brightness of each dot on the screen is made precisely proportional to data stored in the video display memory.

Usually the count data for a radionuclide image are stored on the disk. When the user wants to display an image on the video monitor, the data are transferred to the video display memory (also known as the frame buffer). The display controller then modulates the electron beam intensity according to the data stored in the video memory. The video memory reserves a memory cell for each corresponding raster on the screen, and the number of counts recorded in each memory location determines the raster brightness. The advantages of having a display memory are:

1. It extends the storage capacity of the computer.
2. It allows the CPU to delegate the tedium of continually refreshing the screen to the display controller, thus freeing the CPU for other duties.
3. The video controller can zip data from the video memory to the screen much more effectively than the CPU in retrieving data out of the main memory.

Color Monitors

Color monitors operate using the same principles as monochrome monitors. Instead of having one gun mounted in the rear, there are three (Fig. 3-7). There are triplets of color phosphors called *triads* coated on the glass screen, instead of just one uniform phosphor coating as on a monochrome monitor screen.

Color monitors also have a shadow mask, a metal plate with a number of holes punctured in it, mounted behind the glass screen. Great care is needed when mounting the shadow mask so that each hole in it is precisely aligned opposite a color triad triplet. The shadow mask, acting somewhat like the collimator on a gamma camera, guides the appropriate electron gun to strike the correct color phosphor triad. Different hues are created by varying the intensity of each of the three electron beams passing through the hole in the shadow mask and striking the corresponding color phosphor. The number of colors available on the monitor depends on the number of bits used by the display controller to scale the count data for display. For example, a display controller using 8 bits to scale the number of counts in a pixel can produce 256 different colors.

There are two distinct classes of color monitors: NTSC and RGB. The NTSC color monitors follow the protocol of the NTSC (National Television System Committee) to use one composite video signal to control the electron beam intensity of all three guns. The RGB (Red-Green-Blue) monitors use a separate signal to control each of the three electron guns. The NTSC or composite video monitors produce lower resolution and less well-defined colors in comparison to the RGB monitors, inspiring some lyricists to nickname NTSC monitors as "Never Twice the Same Color" monitors. Because each color on the RGB monitor can be controlled more precisely and no time is spent to decode a composite signal, RGB monitors produce higher resolution graphics, more vividly defined colors, and a faster response than NTSC monitors.

There is a continual debate on whether color monitors or black and white monitors are better suited for presentation of radionuclide

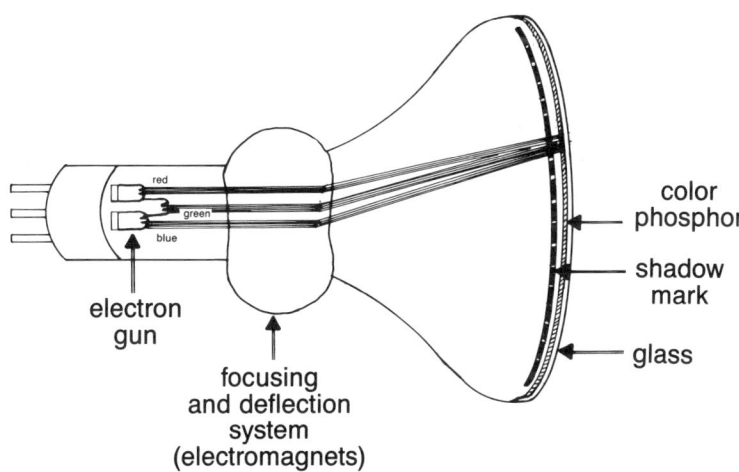

FIGURE 3-7 A color monitor uses three electron guns to activate triplets of color phosphers on the screen.

images. With memory and monitor cost declining rapidly, the economics and esthetics of color display have become more attractive. Some of the newer graphics workstations use color systems having an 8-bit control for each gun, thus allowing 256 levels of intensity for each of the three guns and a total of over 16 million (256 x 256 x 256) colors. For this reason, the argument that color encoding limits the gradation of colors will no longer be valid.

What remains valid for video monitor technology is that monochrome monitors will always produce finer image detail than color monitors. This inherent property is due in part to the narrow electron beam produced by a single electron gun in a monochrome monitor instead of three required by a color monitor. As expected, a small diameter beam produces sharper and smaller rasters on the screen, hence better image resolution. The scanning electron beam in a color monitor will always be larger than that of a monochrome monitor because the beam diameter needs to be large enough to cover the three color phosphor triads. While the resolution of a monochrome monitor is mainly determined by the electron beam diameter, resolution of a color monitor is determined by the number and size of the holes in the shadow mask. In this regard, the effect that the shadow mask has on the resolution of a color video monitor is similar to that of the collimator on a gamma camera. Why? Because the number of rasters and the size of each raster on the display screen depends on the number and size of the holes in the shadow mask as shown in Figure 3-8. The distance between the centers of two holes in the shadow mask is called the dot pitch and is used as an index of the resolution of a color monitor. For example, text characters displayed on a color monitor with a dot pitch of 0.21-0.31 mm appear sharp and continuous, whereas a 0.38-mm or 0.41-mm monitor would show blurred characters with annoying gaps between the dots that make up the characters. Also, the diameter of the electron beam must be larger than the diameter of the hole in the shadow mask in order to cover the color triads adequately.

For both the monochrome and color monitors, good resolution requires a high *bandwidth*, which is the number of rasters struck by the electron beam per second, and is measured in megahertz. Thus, a scanning electron beam that strikes the phosphor surface 16 million times a second is said to have a bandwidth of 16 MHz. The bandwidth of the monitor determines the quality of the image shown

INPUT AND OUTPUT DEVICES 59

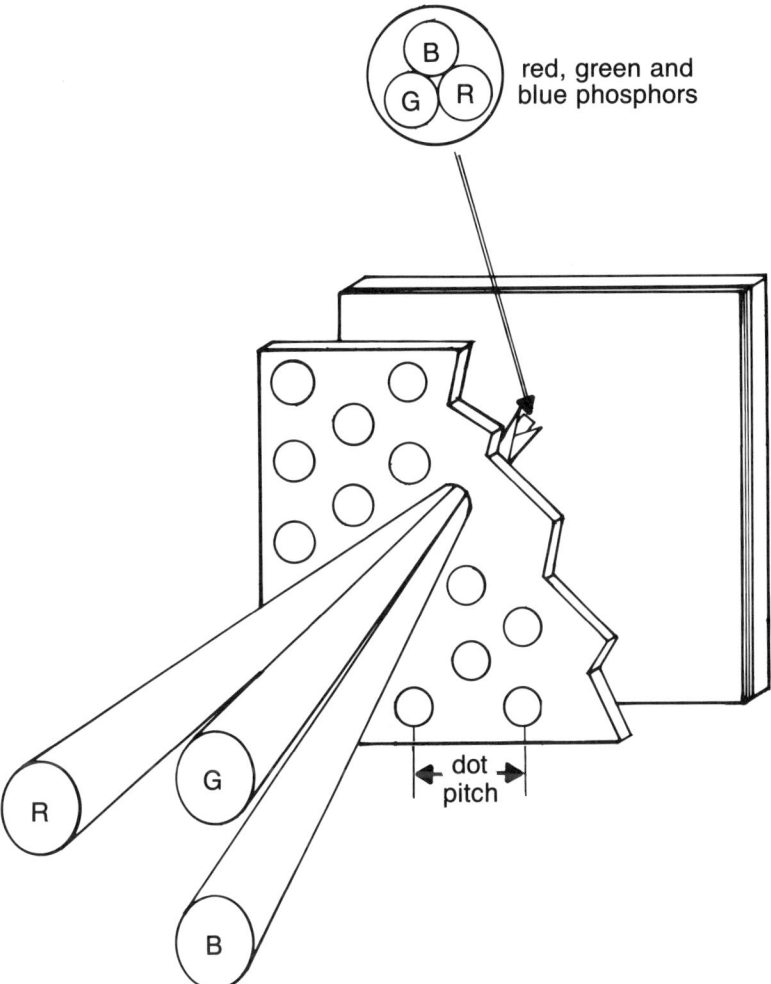

FIGURE 3-8 The shadow mask helps to ensure accurate color production by limiting the electron beams to pass through openings that are aligned precisely with the color triads.

on the screen because it is maximum rate at which the monitor can receive data from the computer. The faster the information is received from the computer, the faster and more sharply the data can be shown on the screen. Commercial television sets have a bandwidth of about 5 MHz. A high quality monitor used for word processing has a bandwidth of 20 MHz, and over 60 MHz for high resolution RGB image displays. Select a monitor whose bandwidth matches that of the computer. You will not gain resolution by having a monitor that is capable of receiving data much faster than the computer can deliver. On the other hand, if the computer can deliver data faster than your monitor can receive it, you will not be getting the maximum possible display resolution.

PRINTERS

Printers play only a minor role in a nuclear medicine computer system in that they serve mainly as a supplementary output device to the CRT terminal by providing a permanent record of the screen display and by presenting graphs, tables, and text in an area much larger than is possible with the usual 12-inch CRT screen. Since radionuclide images constitute the majority of the output data in a nuclear medicine computer system, instant cameras and other film formatters are the principal devices used to record images off the CRT. Printers, if at all present, are used to provide a hardcopy directory of data stored in off-line media, such as the magnetic tapes and optical disks. Until computers are used for other non-image processing functions, such as computerized nuclear medicine reporting systems, printers will continue to be utilized for no more than approximately 1% of the time. A brief description of the variety of printers currently available is offered as an overview.

An imprint on the paper can be made by either *impact* or *nonimpact* printing techniques. The impact printing technique forms an image on paper by striking an inked ribbon against the paper with either a solid font on a daisy wheel or a matrix of pins. Daisy wheel printers produce fully formed characters like those produced by a typewriter, while dot matrix printers produce imprints by matrix pins appearing as an array of dots.

Daisy Wheel Printers

Prior to the advent of laser printers, daisy wheel printers are generically called letter quality printers because the imprints resemble the high quality characters produced by a typewriter in business correspondence. The fully formed characters produced by daisy wheel printers have an attractive appearance and excellent legibility. Daisy wheel printers suffer, however, by being able to offer only about 100 characters on-line, because each character is mechanically made and must be installed as a set in the printer before use. The daisy wheel shows that the available characters are mounted on arms radiating from a hub. When a character is to be printed, a hammer strikes the character element against the inked ribbon and paper in one short stroke and makes an imprint. Characters available to the letter quality printer are limited to the 100 or so typefaces on the daisy wheel. Although a larger number of character sets can be made available by using different daisy wheels, the user has no flexibility to form new characters or symbols, draw curves, or create graphics. Due to the inertia of the massive daisy wheel and the time needed to rotate the desired typeface into position, the speed of a daisy wheel printer is typically limited to about 50 characters per second.

Dot Matrix Printers

The print head on a dot matrix printer consists of a number of pins arranged in one or more vertical rows. The pins are arranged in one vertical column in the 9-pin printheads; the 24-pin printers have three columns of 8-pins arranged in a staggered pattern. Each pin is controlled by a small electromagnet. When an electric current is applied to the solenoid of the electromagnet, a strong magnetic field is created, which propels the pins forward to strike against the ribbon and paper. Current to the solenoid is immediately turned off after the impact, thus collapsing the magnetic field and allowing the pin to spring back to its original position.

As the printhead slides on its track across the width of the paper, the microprocessor inside the printer determines which pins are to be fired to form a vertical slice of the character. Recognizable characters are formed by selectively activating pins in the print head to form a dot pattern such as the 5 x 7 matrix shown in Figure 3-9. Legibility of dot matrix varies depending upon the number of dots used in the array. Characters formed by a matrix of 5 x 7 dots are difficult to read because strokes that should be solid appear broken as the individual dots are distinctly visible. The so-called letter quality printers utilizing printheads with 24 pins are able to create charac-

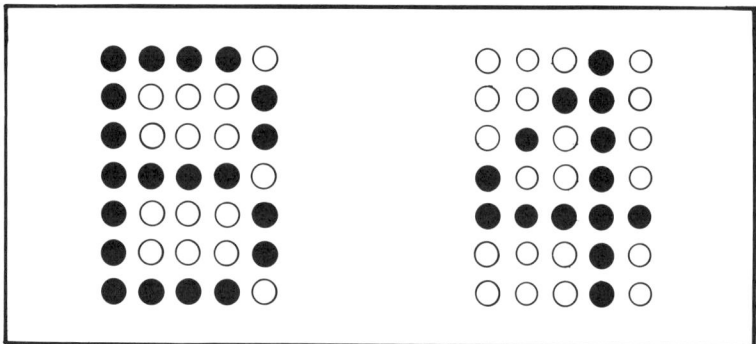

FIGURE 3-9 Dot matrix printers form characters by making an imprint of an array of dots on paper.

ters approaching the quality of daisy wheel printers. Some dot matrix printers produce near letter quality characters by running the print head two or more passes over each character. This printing technique greatly improves the appearance, but this is done at the expense of reduced throughput.

Different fonts, styles, and symbols available to a dot matrix printer are created by software and kept in a ROM inside the printer. Since, the storage capacity of a ROM is much greater than the 100 solid fonts on the spokes of a daisy wheel, dot matrix printers offer a much greater variety of characters on-line than the daisy wheel. By changing one ROM for another, a whole new set of characters becomes available. The user has greater flexibility to plot curves or create special symbols or character styles not already stored in the ROM. The print head of a dot matrix printer weighs much less and does not need to rotate. Hence, printing speeds of 200 cps are common, and speeds in excess of 600 cps can be achieved.

Non-impact printers utilize methods such as ink-jet, electrostatics, heat, and laser to form an image on paper. Some non-impact printers employing dot matrix printing techniques, give low noise and offer high printing speeds in excess of 20,000 lines per minute. The two major limitations of non-impact printers are:

1. They cannot make multiple copies simultaneously.
2. If special chemically-treated paper is required, the operating cost can be considerable, and the printed information

INPUT AND OUTPUT DEVICES

may fade with time. Laser and ink-jet printers offer superior quality prints at moderate printing speeds and have pushed daisy wheel printers into obsolescence.

Laser Printers

Laser printers operate on nearly the same principle as photocopiers. Figure 3-10 shows the elements of a printing engine. A low-power laser under the control of the micro-processor sends short pulses of coherent light to a rotating hexagonal mirror. The light reflecting off the mirror converts portions of the surface of a positively charged drum to negative and creates a latent image. The drum is then sprayed with a positively charged powder called toner which sticks to the negatively charged areas created by the laser. When the paper comes in contact with the drum, the toner image is fused to the paper by heat and pressure. As the paper comes out of the printer, the print drum is cleaned and recharged for the next printing cycle.

The printing speed of laser printers are not only faster than that of daisy wheel printers, but the print quality is much superior. Also,

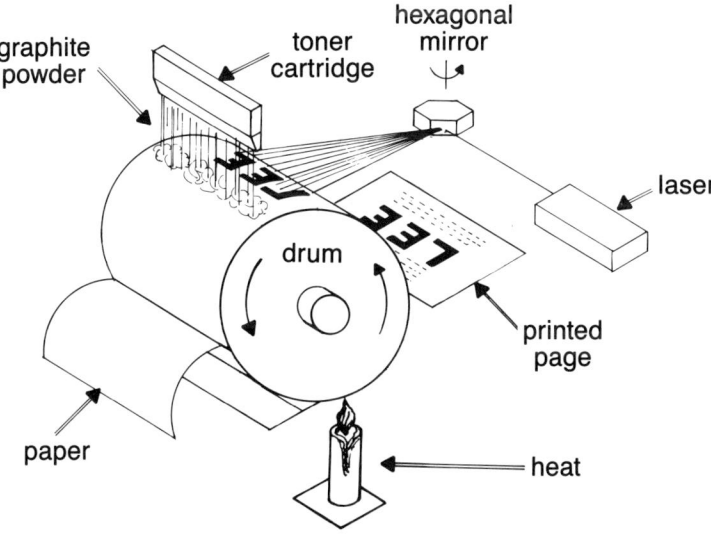

FIGURE 3-10 The printing engine in a laser printer.

the ability of laser printers to produce stunning graphics makes it a fun device for printing reports and brochures—some people call it desktop publishing. Laser printers at this time can only produce black and white images. However, color laser printers soon will be commercially feasible.

Ink-jet Printers

Ink-jet printers are utilized for producing color images on paper. Figure 3-11 shows that the print head of an ink-jet printer can be comprised of several nozzles, each connected to a reservoir of different colored ink. As the array of print heads moves across the paper, jets of ink are sprayed onto the paper under the control of a microprocessor. By shooting fine droplets of colored inks in a sequence as directed by the computer, a high-resolution color image can be formed on the paper.

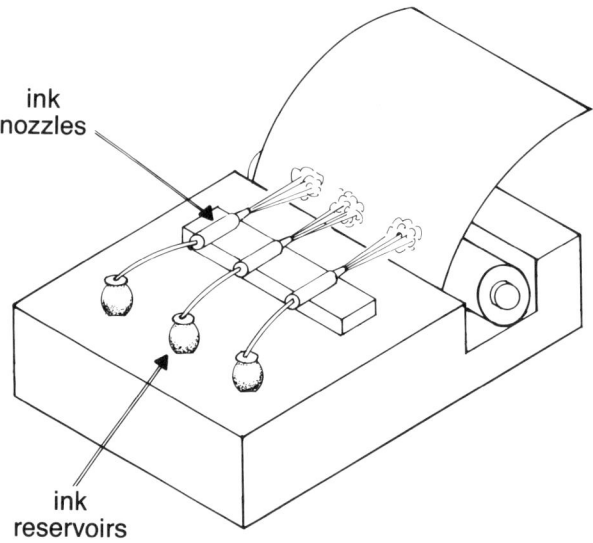

FIGURE 3-11 Ink-jet printers produce color images by spraying fine droplets of color ink on paper.

CONCLUSION

In Chapters 1-3, a short description of the typical hardware components in a nuclear medicine computer system, how each component works, and albeit brief, why they are needed, was provided. All of this powerful computer hardware will serve no purpose unless there are instructions to set it in motion. Computer instructions or software are discussed in the following chapters.

SUGGESTED READINGS FOR CHAPTERS 1-3

1. Bartee T. *Digital computer fundamentals*, sixth edition. New York: McGraw-Hill; 1985.

2. Berke JJ, Ryan B. Gigabytes on-line. *Byte* 1989;14:259-264

3. Bohl M. *Essentials of information processing*. New York: McMillan; 1990.

4. Dessy RE. Choosing a PC: Parts I and II. *Anal Chem* 1986; 58:78-91, 313-333.

5. Fox GC, Paul CM, Advanced computer architecture. *Sci Am* October 1987; 67-74.

6. Jenkins RA. New approaches in parallel computing. *Computers in Physics* 1989; 3:24-32.

7. Kuni CC. Introduction to computers and digital processing. In: *Medical imaging*. Chicago: Yearbook Medical Publishers; 1988.

8. Ryan B. The once and future king—hard disk technology: Reports of its death have been greatly exaggerated. *Byte* 1990;12:301-306.

9. Seitz CL. The cosmic cube. Communications of the ACM, January, 1985.

10. Norton P, Jourdain R. *The hard disk companion.* Brady Books; 1988.

11. Simmons GH, Kereiakes JG, Pickens DR. Computer hardware and software fundamentals. *Radiographics* 1985;5:11-29.

12. Smith AJ. Cache memory design: an evolving art. *IEEE Spectrum* June 1987;46-50.

13. Wiley P. A parallel architecture comes of age at last. *IEEE Spectrum* June, 1987:46-50.

CHAPTER

4

COMPUTER SOFTWARE

INTRODUCTION

The concept of hardware is easy to understand. Hardware are things that we can see and touch and that break down from time to time. The concept of software is more subtle. Software is a set of codes used to instruct the hardware devices on what to do and on when to do it. In the early days of computers, instructions were entered into the computer by manually flipping an array of switches on the control console. As computers became more sophisticated, symbolic codes replaced switch flipping as the means of instructing the computer.

These codes are usually typed into the computer via the keyboard. If we consider each key on the keyboard as a push button, instead of a typewriter key, the notion of software is more easily understood. Each time we press a key on the keyboard, we act as though we are pushing a button on the computer control console. Each push of a button will cause a certain hardware component to do something. Typing a list of symbolic codes on the keyboard is equivalent to pushing a series of buttons, in a unique sequence, to trigger different parts of the computer system to act in a predetermined fashion. A *computer program* is a particular sequence of symbolic codes, which causes the computer hardware to perform a defined task. The generic term *software* refers to any computer program used to manipulate the operation of the computer.

TYPES OF COMPUTER SOFTWARE

The first lesson to be learned about computer software is that there are a myriad of types; each acts at a different level in the hierarchy of computer operations. At the lowest level, a long series of instructions may do nothing more than turn on a particular switch. A single keystroke at the highest level of command may be all that is necessary to trigger the computer to reconstruct transverse axial images from the projection images. Basically, software comprises three categories:

1. Application software
2. System control software
3. Programming software.

These categories are by no means standard classifications. They are merely an arbitrary creation for explaining the methodology of computer software.

Application software acts at the highest level in the computer operations. In a nuclear medicine computer system, the application software consist of programs for data acquisition and manipulation. One example of an application program, or software, is a sequence of instructions for smoothing a radionuclide image. The clinical software package that comes with each nuclear medicine computer system is a collection of application programs which enable us to acquire and process the radionuclide data in a variety of ways. The principles for some of the application programs used for acquisition and processing of images are discussed in later chapters.

System control software includes the *operating system* (OS) and a host of *utility programs*. An operating system is a collection of recipe programs that literally tells the computer how to operate. The OS interprets the request made by the user, or the application program, and then invokes the proper hardware to carry out the requested task. Without the OS, you would be forced to communicate with the computer using zeroes and ones, instead of simple mnemonics such as "Copy." In short, an operating system is a master program that controls the overall operation of a computer. It acts as a liaison between the user, the application program, and all the different gadgets inside the computer. It is the first program you call upon when you turn on the computer, and the last program to terminate when you turn off the computer.

Utility programs are also called *system utilities*. They are application programs which make the life of a programmer easier by filling in the gaps left by the OS, a programming language, or even another application program. Many people consider system utilities an extension to the OS because they perform their duties at the operating system level. For example, a utility program might keep a directory of data on a Winchester disk, transfer data from one disk to another, or allow the computer to do other work while a data file is being printed. Programming software is a set of instructions codes (called programming language) that the computer understands and translates into actions. All application programs, operating systems, and system utilities are written using one or more programming languages. There are literally hundreds of different programming languages developed since the birth of digital computers in the mid-1940s. They vary from the simple mnemonics that represents zeros and ones to those with English-like commands. However, only about a dozen or so of these languages have found widespread use. The section on programming software provides a brief overview of commonly used programs and highlights their purpose, similarities, advantages, and disadvantages.

OPERATING SYSTEM

An OS can be called a master program or a slave program, depending on which part of the operating system you refer to. In either case, the OS acts as a messenger between the user and the computer. The user sees the computer as a powerful machine that can be commanded to do useful work utilizing its many resources. These resources can be application programs, data of various kinds, and a variety of hardware devices. The fundamental function of an OS is to take commands from the user, determine its meaning, and then invoke the necessary software and hardware devices to fulfill the requested services. As you can imagine, putting a computer to work means controlling and manipulating millions of switches and instruction codes repetitively, which is both boring and tedious and certainly not an easy task for the human user. The OS is a large complicated program that acts as a "pretty face," linking the computer and the user (Fig. 4-1). It accepts a short and easy to remember command from the user, and then shields the user from the tedious work while it performs the assigned task at the hardware level. The ability to request hardware and software services simply and conveniently maximizes the utilization of the computer's power. The standardized ways to utilize the resources of a computer also accelerate the development of new software.

Of the many functions performed by the OS, many of them can be classified into one of the following three categories:

1. Command and program execution function.
2. Input/output (I/O) control.
3. File management.

The following example illustrates these three classifications. The first thing to do after power is turned on is to bring up the computer, i.e., put the computer in the ready mode for accepting com-

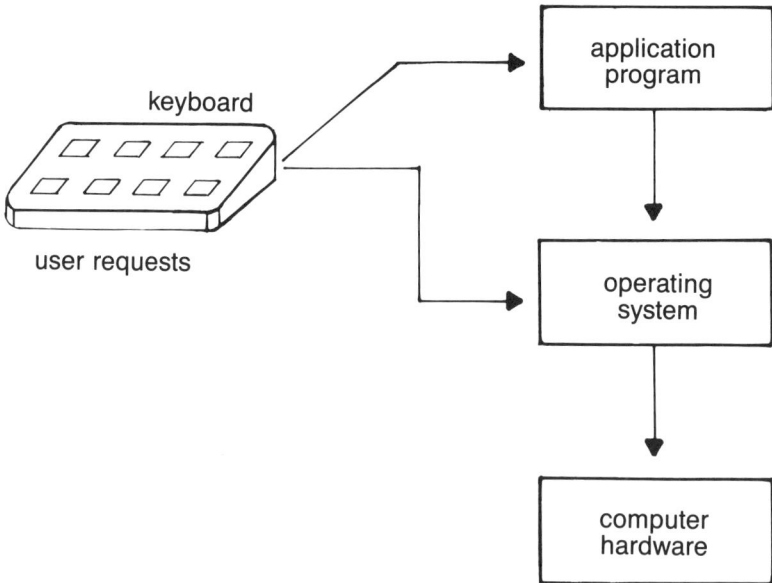

FIGURE 4-1 The OS acts as the servant between the user's requests and the computer hardware.

mands from the user. As discussed in Chapter 1, the process of bringing the computer up into a running condition is called *bootstrapping* or simply *boot,* which is computer jargon for loading and starting the execution of the OS. In every computer there is a short program consisting of only a few instructions stored in a read only memory (ROM). Once the computer is on, this short program in the ROM immediately activates the sequence of loading the OS from a magnetic tape or more commonly from a disk. An OS usually takes up much more space than is available in the CPU memory. During bootstrapping only a portion of the OS is loaded into the CPU memory, and that part of the OS remains active as long as the power to the computer stays on. Portions of the OS that are not in the CPU memory are kept on the disk. Any part of the OS on the disk can be loaded into the CPU memory when its service is needed. This type of operating system is referred to as a disk operating system (DOS).

When the computer is up and running you will see a system prompt, represented by a question mark, a blinking cursor, or some peculiar symbol, which means "what can I do for you?" Answering the prompt, with a command or the name of a program, initiates a search by the OS for the proper program to execute.

A command usually refers to a program within the OS itself, while a program refers to an application program outside the OS. One of the functions of the OS is to differentiate names entered by the user as OS commands or application program names, and then search for it in the proper location in the memory or on disk. If the command or program is found residing on the disk, the OS then allocates space in the CPU memory to store the instructions for the system command or application program.

In the 1950s and the mid-1960s, computers typically operated in the *batch mode* to serve a large number of users. In a typical *run,* the computer operator collected programs on punched cards or tapes from a number of users. A batch of the collected programs were then fed into the computer all at once. These programs were first routed by the OS to a mass storage device, such as a disk or a magnetic tape, to await their turn for execution. These programs were then executed individually, in succession, thereby reducing the delay from stopping the computer and manually loading the programs one at a time.

In the mid-1960s *time-sharing* OSs were developed, which allowed a large number of people to utilize a powerful central computer facility. In the time-sharing mode, the computer can work on two or more tasks concurrently. In reality, a computer can only do one job at a time. However, the CPU usually finishes its assigned task in a fraction of a second. Most of its time is spent waiting for input from the user, for the printer to finish printing, for the disk to find the data, or for the monitor to display an image, and so forth. A time-sharing OS redirects the CPU during these unproductive periods to work on other tasks instead of merely waiting. The CPU cannot execute two programs simultaneously. However, the operating system switches the attention of the computer so rapidly from one job to the other that the computer appears to be executing several programs simultaneously. A time-sharing OS therefore has the responsibility to keep track of where each program is located in memory, at which point in each program that the CPU last exited, and to be constantly on the lookout for any idle time of the CPU.

The time-sharing OS was an important development because it greatly increased the efficiency of the computer by reducing its idle time. Additionally, a computer in the time-sharing mode allows remotely located people to get access to the computer conveniently via a terminal and a telephone modem. For a computer with a great many users, the illusion of instant access to the computer can evaporate very fast during the busy part of the day. The CPU in the time-sharing mode serves each user in a round-robin manner. It goes from one job to another only when a pause occurs. When the computer is in demand by a number of users, each user has to sit patiently in front of the terminal for his turn to be served. When a person just sits to wait for the computer to respond, minutes seem like hours, especially if he is paying toll on the telephone call.

Mini-computers of the 1970s extended the time-sharing concept into the *real-time* OS. In time-sharing systems, every user has a slice of the time pie with relatively equal priority as far as being served by the CPU. A real-time OS, on the other hand, assigns priorities according to the type of requests. A request to start the acquisition of a radionuclide image from the gamma camera, for example, has a higher priority than a request to display an image that has previously been acquired. A real-time OS is important to a nuclear medicine computer system because certain time-dependent tasks, such as acquiring counts from a first-pass nuclear cardiology study, must be done as rapidly as possible at the time the event is taking place. Therefore, all other operations cannot have priority over such a task. The so-called foreground/background operation is a simple type of real-time OS. The program running in the foreground has a higher priority than the one in the background. Keep in mind that a job always takes longer to finish, whether the computer is running in time-sharing or real-time mode, when compared to batch processing. Even though acquisition has top priority in any nuclear medicine computer system, if the CPU is busy when an event occurs in the gamma camera, it cannot immediately abandon whatever it is doing at that moment and record the count. Consequently that particular count will be lost, and the acquisition time then lengthens for the given preset count. In case the acquisition is terminated by a preset time, as is the situation with dynamic studies, fewer counts will be recorded if another program is running simultaneously.

The first OSs were created to assist with the input and output functions of the computer. A conceptually simple task such as printing a line of text may require writing over a dozen lines in a lower-level language such as machine or assembly language. By having a set of I/O functions available in the OS at all times, the programmer does not need to divert his attention from problem-solving to taking care of the uninteresting I/O operations, thus drastically reducing the tedium and the number of steps needed to write a program.

File management, an exotic term which includes chores such as storing data or programs on the disk, formatting a blank disk, and maintaining a directory on the disk, is another important duty of the OS. Unfortunately, every OS performs these functions differently. Thus, a computer may not be able to read a disk full of useful data or programs that have been recorded by another computer running under a different OS. In fact, operating systems are proprietary programs written by a vendor to manipulate the overall operation of their hardware devices. A few OSs are slowly becoming the de facto standards because there are many computers that use that OS or because the features in that OS are so attractive that the users voluntarily adopt it into their computers.

In summary, the OS provides a collection of programs needed by nearly all software, so that the programmer does not need to reinvent the wheel with each new application program. Coordinating the actions between the software and hardware, and managing the resources in the computer system are among the essential functions of the OS.

PROGRAMMING SOFTWARE

Low-Level Computer Programming Languages

A low-level language is a set of instruction codes, which correspond closely to the operations that are carried out by a particular computer. A low-level language is comprised of codes that the computer can act on directly. On the other hand, high-level languages are relatively machine independent and must be translated to the native language of the computer before any action can take place. However, low-level languages are cumbersome to use; hence, they are mostly used in situations where high-level languages are inefficient or impossible to take command of the special features of a given machine. For example, programs to control and communicate with peripheral devices such as the printer and disk drive are usually written in a low-level language because they require special instructions that are not available in a high-level language and speed is critical. Unlike the large variety of high-level languages, low-level languages mainly consist of the machine and assembly languages.

Machine Language

Regardless of which language a person selects to write his program, the program is ultimately translated to the one language that a computer can understand, the binary zeroes and ones. Every CPU contains a built-in set of instruction codes represented by groups of zeroes and ones. Remember that an instruction code on the hardware level is represented by a unique sequence of **On** and **Off** switches. These binary codes represent the actual instructions the computer understands and works. The CPU will perform specific operations in response to the presentation of a specific binary pattern. Because the electronic circuitry of a computer is ultimately controlled by the **On** or **Off** states of specific switches, any application program must eventually be translated in terms of these binary patterns. For this reason, binary codes form what is known as machine lanaguage.

Usually each manufacturer defines their own set of instruction codes and features into machine language in order to take advantage of their specific hardware design and the intended applications of the CPU. Furthermore, there is no standardization among manufacturers as to the binary code, even for common functions such as addition and subtraction. Unless a manufacturer purposely incorporates the instruction set of another manufacturer into his own CPU, any two different computers will most likely have two completely different machine languages. This means that a program written in machine language for one computer is unlikely to run on a computer made by a different manufacturer.

The major reason why some rudimentary programs are still written in machine language is because a machine language program will run faster. There are several obvious disadvantages with writing programs directly in machine language. Writing a program in machine language is extremely tedious and prone to error. To write a program as simple as adding two numbers together requires the programmer to look up the number code in zeroes and ones for about 10 different operations. The machine has no problem in distinguishing 1010101001 from 0110101001 and remembers what each code requires it to do. For most mortal programmers, however, the string of zeroes and ones will dazzle the eyes very soon, and a misplaced zero or one becomes very difficult to detect. Besides, the function of the heap of zeroes and ones is far from obvious and *debugging* (computerese for finding and correcting errors in a computer program) is not an easy task. For these reasons, machine language is rarely used to write anything but the simplest and most speed-critical programs.

Assembly Language

Assembly language was developed to avoid writing each machine instruction directly into binary codes. Assembly language utilizes *mnemonics,* a short word or abbreviation representing a series of binary codes for each machine operation. Programming with assembly language is more convenient because the English words or abbreviations used for the mnemonics give hints as to what the computer hardware is to do, obviating the need to constantly look up the binary number codes. The use of mnemonics thus greatly reduces the frequency of entering a wrong machine code. Also, an assembly language program requires fewer steps than an equivalent program written in machine language. All the above features make an assembly language program easier to understand and easier to debug than one written in machine language.

Because computers can only understand instructions in zeroes and ones, a program written in assembly language must be translated into binary code before it can be executed. The word *execute* in the computer literature means the actual carrying out of an instruction by the computer. The process of translating an assembly language into machine language is called *assembly*. When assembly language was first used for programming, translation was done by hand. The programmer wrote the program in assembly language and then translated each mnemonic into machine language by looking up a table for the corresponding binary codes. Because this translation step is highly mechanical, it can be carried out by the computer itself. To have the computer perform the translation, a program called an *assembler* must first be *loaded* into the computer memory. The term *load* is a software buzz-word for entering and storing a program or data into the computer memory. The application program (in assembly language) is then loaded into the computer. After the complete assembly program has been entered, the assembler is then executed to convert the mnemonics into the corresponding binary machine language code.

The above discussion on translating an assembly language program into a machine language program illustrates that there is still a one-to-one correspondence between a mnemonic and a binary machine instruction code. To write an assembly program, the programmer is still required to know the hardware structure of the computer and to write an instruction code in mnemonics for every step the computer has to perform. Therefore, assembly language programs also tend to be quite long.

Even though the meaning of a mnemonic is easier to remember than binary codes, assembly language is still tied closely to the computer's primitive language than to the natural language used by the programmer in his thought process. Because computers only do what they are told to do rather than what the programmer wants them to do, each individual instruction must be included in the program. If one minute step is left out, the end result will not be what the programmer intended, hence the program is said to have a bug.

Nevertheless, assembly language continues to be the language of choice for a number of applications. First, many time-critical portions of large application programs are written in assembly language because it is faster than high-level languages, which are discussed in the next section. Second, assembly language allows direct control of the functions for all of the hardware devices in a computer. For example, in some software packages for nuclear medicine, a number of programs utilize *routines* in assembly language for the acquisition, display and manipulation of the radionuclide images. A routine is a program segment written to do a certain specific functions. A number of routines are kept in a section of the software package called the routine library, which can be called to service by a main program at any time. Another attractive quality of assembly language is that many machine-specific instructions are more efficiently handled in assembly language; thus they can be linked to a high-level language program to improve execution efficiency.

High-Level Computer Programming Languages

Whereas machine and assembly languages are called low-level or machine-oriented languages, high-level languages are called problem-oriented languages. The person developing a program using a low-level language needs to be constantly aware of how each processing step is being handled by the computer. The so-called high-level languages were developed to help programmers concentrate on the concepts needed to solve their problems without having to be concerned about the inner-working mechanisms of their computing machine. These high-level languages allow the programmer to communicate with the computer using English language words and notations similar to standard mathematical nomenclatures, with only a few rules governing the usage of the language. The rules of a high-level language are called the *syntax*. Each instruction in a high-level language is called a statement, rather than an instruction code, in order to emphasize its close resemblance to English statements.

Programs developed using a high-level language are more compact than those written in machine or assembly language. One statement in a high level language can take the place of a number of assembly language codes. These features make high-level language programs shorter, less prone to error, and easier to understand and debug. Furthermore, such programs are less dependent on the machine, so that a program written in a high-level language on one computer can be run on another computer without having to undergo major modifications.

FORTRAN

Dozens of high-level languages have been developed over the years. However, the language with the most profound influence on the development of other high-level languages was FORTRAN. FORTRAN (FORmula TRANslation) was developed in the mid-1950s to perform scientific and numerical calculations and is still widely used today for those purposes. FORTRAN is cumbersome, if not virtually useless, for processing text information such as reports. While FORTRAN relieves the programmer from worrying about the details of machine operation and instruction codes, it also imposes a number of arbitrary constraints on the use of language. For example, the letters I through N are reserved for representing integers, numbers without a decimal fraction. The most serious deficiencies of FORTRAN are its awkward method of controlling the execution sequence of the program statements and its lack of modularity. However, we must keep in mind that FORTRAN was developed in the mid-1950s for mathematicians and scientists to perform lengthy but straightforward numerical calculations. As the experience and ideas for computer utilization grew, so grew the demand on the flexibility and power of the programming language. That is why a number of high-level languages have been developed to overcome some of the limitations of FORTRAN. In fact, FORTRAN has undergone many changes. The more modern version, FORTRAN 77, has incorporated many new ideas of program design such as the top-down structural approach, features for graphics, and more convenient methods for handling input/output operations of non-numeric data.

COBOL

COBOL (Common Business Oriented Languages) was developed shortly after FORTRAN to accommodate descriptive text information, but contained only limited capacity for numerical computations. Thus, COBOL found very little use in the scientific community. However, it is widely used by business organizations for keeping transaction records, alphabetic data files, and document preparation. The main reason for the popularity of COBOL in the commercial field is that it contains the vocabulary of the business establishment. Unlike most symbolic programming languages, the syntax of COBOL conforms more to English grammar than the notations of mathematics and logic. Therefore, the program instructions are so easy to understand that even a beginner with no background in computer programming can comprehend the meaning.

PL/1

FORTRAN and COBOL complemented each other as to the needs of scientific and business programming well into the mid-1960s. By that time, business users wanted to utilize the computer for economic modelling, statistics, business forecasting, operation research (a mathematical method for optimizing a business activity under known or assumed constraints), and so on. At the same time, scientists wanted to simplify the sorting, editing, and input/output operation of both numeric and especially non-numeric data.

For these reasons, the language of PL/1 (Programming Language/One) was developed. The thrust behind PL/1 was to develop an all-purpose language that would satisfy both numeric and non-numeric applications. PL/1 was also designed as a versatile language to be used by both beginning programmers and as well as experts, merging together the salient points of COBOL and FORTRAN. PL/1 permits program statements to develop into modules, instead of one long list of statements. This new feature is well suited for structured programming techniques as advocated by computer scientists.

Although PL/1 was implemented on a number of different computers and for many years was taught as an introductory programming course for students at many universities, it failed to gain acceptance as an universal language. One message was clearly seen from this ambitious effort: special application needs, programming techniques, and programmer personalities are diverse. An "all-purpose" language remains an elusive goal for the creators of computer language.

Pascal

Pascal, developed in the late 1960s by Niklus Wirth of Zurich, Switzerland and named after the French mathematician Blaise Pascal, is another milestone in the genealogy of computer language. It was originally developed for teaching the concept of *structured programming,* which is a modern idea of top-down program design, emphasizing the planning of the program's main objectives first with attention to the details later. The structured approach forces the programmer to think in terms of larger conceptual units; thus, it keeps one's mind on the forest instead of the individual trees.

The structure of a program using the top-down design is much like that of a pyramid. The program is built upon a number of modules, called "procedures" in Pascal. In the planning stage, we should only concern ourselves with what each module or procedure is to do and not with how it performs the job. After we have decided what each procedure should do, then we can work out the minute details within each procedure so it is able to accomplish its assigned task. If we decide to change the function of a given procedure, the modification should not involve a large number of changes in other procedures. Therefore, a well-designed program should consist of a number of relatively independent modules.

Pascal contains a number of built-in procedures for mathematical and logical decision-making functions. The manipulation of alphabetic data is just as convenient as the handling of numbers. In short, Pascal has some of the power of FORTRAN and PL/1, but possesses greater flexibility and modularity. In fact, it is easier for a novice to learn Pascal than FORTRAN, PL/1, or COBOL.

It should be emphasized that Pascal is not the panacea for solving all of our programming problems. It has been received with great enthusiasm because people discovered how easy it is to learn, read and write, and modify a Pascal program. However, Pascal was developed as a tool to teach the concept of structured programming, not as a general-purpose programming language. There are many intentional omissions so that the student can concentrate on the gist of the programming technique.

Pascal is considered a milestone because the structured approach has proven to be an effective method for software development; it is taught and emphasized at all levels of programming. More significantly, Pascal inspired the development of a whole new genera-

COMPUTER SOFTWARE

tion of programming languages based on the principles of top-down, modular, and structured approach.

Ada

The much talked about-language that is still under development at the time of this writing is Ada, which is the most recent attempt to develop an all-purpose language by the Department of Defense. The syntax and construct of Ada are based largely on Pascal, except that the language is much more complex. The complexity shown by preliminary versions of Ada have led to the pessimistic prediction that people will only learn Ada to do mission-critical projects with the military, not because of the attractiveness of the language. However, there is also hope that with greater familiarity with this potentially powerful language, applications unforeseen at this time may be developed.

BASIC

Basic (Beginner's All-purpose Symbolic Instruction Codes), originally developed to enable students (liberal art and science majors) to quickly learn the principles of computer programming, is a major breakthrough which takes the mystery out of computer programming. Because of BASIC the programmer no longer has to worry about such details as the idiosyncrasies of computer hardware, the address location of a variable in the computer memory, how to format the printout, or how the arithmetic is performed. BASIC language performs these chores automatically for the programmer.

At the time BASIC was developed, the prevalent practice was for the programmer to write his program initially with paper and pencil. When he was satisfied with the program on paper, the program statements were then punched on cards or paper tape and handed to the computer operator to feed into the computer along with other programs. This type of computer operation was called *batch processing*. The turn around time was slow, especially in organizations with a large number of users. In case an error was detected in the program, the programmer had to go through the whole cycle again, with much delay and frustration to get the program done and running correctly. One of the major contributions BASIC makes to computer programming is the implementation of a high-level language to work with the new *time-sharing* concept on large-scale computers.

BASIC is an interactive language. It allows the programmer to work more directly with the computer. When a mistake is encountered during execution, the computer stops and informs the programmer that at a certain point in the program an error was found. The programmer can make the correction and then continue on with the execution of the rest of the program. A BASIC program can be made to pause and ask the user to enter data directly into the computer terminal. This type of *user-friendliness*—an over-used term nowadays—was unheard of during the days of "user too-bad" batch processing.

Like Pascal, the worldwide use of BASIC, especially for microcomputers, has gone beyond the expectation of the language originators. Although BASIC is rarely used for writing nuclear medicine software, it is widely used in personal computers because it can be squeezed into as little as 8 KB of computer memory and is probably the easiest language to learn. However, along with these advantages, BASIC does have drawbacks. BASIC is not a structured language, so a long program can be very difficult to debug or modify. BASIC programs also run slower than an equivalent program in other high-level languages such as FORTRAN, PL/1, and Pascal.

C

If we refer to machine and assembly languages as low-level languages, and FORTRAN, COBOL, PL/1, BASIC and Pascal as high-level languages, then C ought to be called a mid-level language. C, a concise language with a vocabulary of only 30 reserved words, was developed for seasoned programmers, not novices. A C program can be difficult to understand unless the programmer takes great time or discipline in entering the program statements into the computer in a readable style. Pascal and BASIC, which assume that the programmer is wrong more often than not, contains a wealth of built-in features to check for errors. Unlike them, C takes the view that the professional programmer knows all the rules of the language. When goofs occur, these "high priests" of computer programming can debug the program without the computer telling them the type and location of the errors. However, many new versions of C have been appearing with extensive facilities to ease the pain of debugging. Nevertheless, the burden of error detection still rests heavily on the programmer.

There are several reasons why C is the language of choice for complex software projects, in spite of it being more difficult to use than other high-level languages. For example, many graphics and animation sequences in film (e.g., the now classic science fiction movies, "Return of the Jedi" and "Star Wars") are created using C because C programs are compact, thus obviating the need for a large CPU memory for long and complex programs. The trend in new application software development is to make the programs easy to use. These user-friendly programs tend to be large and complex so that the user can be rescued from most common mistakes. The compactness of C thus makes it the language of choice for the new generation of software, not only for nuclear medicine but also for such diverse fields as business and the arts.

Another reason is C's highly transportable characteristics. C programs can be developed on one computer and run on another, and still can take advantage of the peculiarities and subtleties of the hardware features of that computer. Because C programs are not tied to any particular computer and because they are executed at a speed close to that of assembly-language programs, C has been called a *portable-assembly language.* C has included in it many of the advanced structured programming features found in Pascal, which are recognized by many professional programmers. Already, C has become the language in many of the nuclear medicine software running on the 32-bit computers.

There are many more programming languages that I have not even mentioned. The conclusion you have probably reached is that there is no one ideal language. Each language has its own advantages and disadvantages. The development of a universal language is still to come. New languages will continually be developed to address special purposes and needs. With the current state-of-the-art, we select a language that will best fulfill our application needs.

Implementation of a High-Level Language

Just as the use of assembly language requires an assembler program to translate the mnemonics into machine codes, all high- or mid-level languages similarly require a special program to translate the program statements into machine codes. An *implementation* is such a program, converting the high-level language notations into an equivalent series of machine instruction codes.

The implementation of a language can be classified as either an *interpreter* or a *compiler*. An interpreter translates each program statement into machine codes as the program is executed; the machine codes are not saved in the computer memory. The interpreter translates one statement at a time and executes them as it goes along, without creating an equivalent program in binary codes in the computer memory. Therefore, the interpreter must be present in the computer memory at all times while the high-level language program is being executed.

A compiler, on the other hand, translates each statement of the entire program into machine codes in one continuous step. The machine codes are not executed as they are produced. Instead, the equivalent machine codes for each statement are saved in the computer memory to form an *object program*—the equivalent program in machine language. The object program can be executed only after the compilation is completed. Keep in mind that the program to be executed later is the object program in machine language, not the original program in high-level language. The object program can be transferred and stored onto a disk or tape for later execution. Therefore, the compiler need not be present in the computer memory when the object program is being executed.

The term compiler may sound strange, but it is actually very descriptive of its translation process. The compiler is a large computer program that contains tables of machine instructions in zeroes and ones for the corresponding words and symbols in a high-level language. During the translation process, the compiler looks up the equivalent binary codes for each program statement, and stacks them up in the computer memory. At the end of the translation process, a complete object program is compiled—or piled up—in the computer's memory. The object program contains exactly the same instructions as the original high-level language program, except that it is given in machine language. The object program can be run immediately after compilation because it is saved in the memory. The object program can also be saved on disk for execution later. Since the object program is already in machine language, the compiler need not be present during execution.

A high-level language can be implemented in either the compiled or interpreted form. Traditionally, however, certain languages usually appear in one form or the other. FORTRAN, COBOL, Pascal, and C are generally compiled. Although BASIC is almost synonymous with interpreted languages, compiled versions of BASIC are also available and widely used.

The main advantage of a compiled language over an interpreted language is faster execution speed. Every time a statement in an interpreted language is executed, the interpreter must translate it into a proper sequence of machine codes. If a statement is repeatedly executed, say 30 times for instance, the statement must be repetitiously translated 30 times, which is time-consuming. In the case of a compiled language, the statements need to go through translation only once, no matter how many times they are executed. A compiled program thus runs much faster than an interpreted version.

For program development, the interactive nature of interpreted language allows the programmer to stop program execution at any time, for debugging or inserting new statements, and then continue on with the execution, including the latest corrections. These convenient features of an interpreted language make progamming easier. On the other hand, anytime a modification has to be made in a program during compilation, such as correcting a typographical mistake near the end of a long program, it is a frustrating process for the programmer. To make such a correction, the programmer must exit from the compiler, call up an editing program to make the modification, and then call up the compiler to re-compile the program once again from the very beginning.

CONCLUSION

By focusing the discussion on the principles of the OS and the characteristics of programming languages, I hope that readers now have a good understanding of the concepts of computer programming and will not be mystified by jargon that too often "pops up" in the literature. Furthermore, these basic software groups are not only the foundation for the image acquisition and processing software to be discussed in the ensuing chapters, but they are also the tools for the development of every imaginable piece of software (e.g., accounting, education, games, robotics, etc.).

SUGGESTED READINGS

1. Denning PJ, Brown RL. Operating systems. *Sci Am* 1984; 252:94-106.

2. Kay A. Computer software. *Sci Am* 1984;252:53-59.

3. Tesler LG. Programming languages. *Sci Am* 1984;252:70-78.

4. Weselblat RL. *History of programming languages.* New York: Academic Press; 1981.

CHAPTER

5

NUCLEAR MEDICINE IMAGE ACQUISITION METHODS

INTRODUCTION

The operating system and the different programming languages are software tools for the writing of application programs. Application programs, which refer to computer programs written to accomplish certain specific tasks, are different from algorithms. An algorithm is a conceptual method for solving a problem, while a program is a set of instructions to the computer for carrying out the algorithm.

The software package in each nuclear medicine computer system contains a number of programs for collecting image data from the gamma camera, and an even greater number of programs for processing the collected image data to extract information for patient management.

METHODS OF DATA ACQUISITION

The input data to a nuclear medicine computer are mostly counts collected from the gamma camera during the course of a radionuclide study. For every photon emitted from the radionuclide within the patient and entering the gamma camera, three electrical pulses are produced. Two of the pulses represent the coordinates of the photon interaction site in the plane of the NaI crystal. The third pulse represents the energy of the incident photon. If this energy falls within the window of the pulse-height analyzer, a pulse, or the unblank signal in gamma camera terminology, is produced. The pulse turns on the electron beam in the cathode ray tube of the gamma camera so that a spot of light will be produced on the screen phosphor in accordance with the coordinates of the scintillation event in the NaI crystal.

Since signals produced by the gamma camera are analog in nature, they must first be converted to an equivalent binary signal using the analog-to-digital converter (ADC) before they can be understood by the computer. The pulse from the gamma camera is used as a trigger to inform the ADC converter that a pair of signals needs to be transformed for input to the computer. Once the analog-to-digital conversion is done, the count is entered into the computer memory by one of the two following data acquisition methods: (1) the frame mode or (2) the list mode.

FRAME-MODE ACQUISITION

Frame mode is the principal method of recording counts from the gamma camera to produce a radionuclide image. To demonstrate this method of data acquisition, imagine that a block of computer memory is laid out in a square mosaic circumscribing the field of view of the gamma camera as in Figure 5-1. The square mosaic commonly consists of 64 x 64, 128 x 128, or 256 x 256 picture elements (pixels). Thus, there are 4K, 16K, and 64K pixels forming one radionuclide image, respectively. Such a square mosaic is commonly called an *image matrix, image array,* or *pixel array.*

Each pixel in the image matrix has a one-to-one correspondence with a given location in the plane of the NaI crystal. For every scintillation event that produces a signal acceptable to the pulse-height analyzer, the number of counts in the pixel corresponding to the coordinates of the scintillation site is incremented by one. If a 64 x 64 matrix is circumscribing a gamma camera having a 40-cm diameter field of view, then each pixel in the image matrix covers an area of 6.25 x 6.25 mm (400 mm/64 pixels = 6.25 mm/pixel) on the face of the camera. For a 128 x 128 matrix covering the same 40-cm diameter field of view, each pixel provides a resolution of 3.1 x 3.1 mm (400 mm/128 pixels = 3.13 mm/pixel). Thus, the spatial resolution of the computer image is increased as the number of pixels in the image matrix is increased.

IMAGE ACQUISITION METHODS

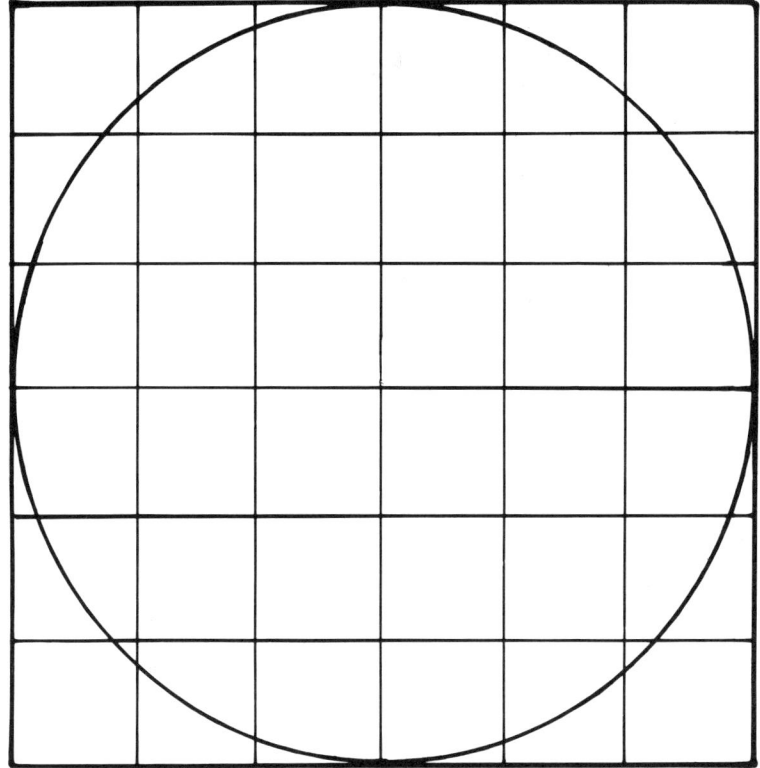

FIGURE 5-1 In frame-mode acquisition an array of pixels is superimposed on the imaging area of the gamma camera. Each pixel is actually an unique storage location in the computer memory that record counts from a designated portion of the NaI crystal.

However, as the number of pixels in an image matrix is increased, the number of counts stored in each pixel of the larger matrix must be increased as well so that the statistical noise is not raised concomitantly. Figure 5-2A shows a 2 x 2 image matrix with 444 counts in each pixel, and this number of counts gives a percentage standard deviation (% s.d.) of 4.6% ($100\%\sqrt{444}$) in each pixel. Since all four pixels have an equal number of counts, we say there are no hot or cold defects in the image. In Figure 5-2B the hot spot obscured in the 2 x 2 matrix is readily seen in the middle of the 4 x 4 matrix. Thus, the 4 x 4 image matrix yields a higher spatial resolution, even though both matrices contain the same number of counts. However, the statistical noise in each pixel as measured by the percentage standard deviation is about twice as high. In this example, the number of counts acquired into the 4 x 4 matrix should be quadrupled in order to maintain the same statistical noise level as in the 2 x 2 matrix. As a rule, the number of counts acquired to form an image should be quadrupled whenever the dimensions of an image array are doubled. In practice this rule is seldom exercised because of the excessive imaging time involved. In fact, the number of counts acquired into the matrix is increased at the most

A

100	100	100	100
100	144	144	100
100	144	144	100
100	100	100	100

number of counts
in each pixel

10	10	10	10
10	8.3	8.3	10
10	8.3	8.3	10
10	10	10	10

% noise in
each pixel $\dfrac{100\%}{\sqrt{N}}$

B

444	444
444	444

number of counts
in each pixel

4.6	4.6
4.6	4.6

% noise in
each pixel $\dfrac{100\%}{\sqrt{N}}$

FIGURE 5-2 The hot spot at the center of the 4 x 4 image matrix (A) is obscured in the 2 x 2 matrix (B). Thus, resolution of the digitized image is improved when using a large image matrix.

by a factor of two, when the matrix dimensions are doubled. In so doing, higher statistical noise is the trade-off for better spatial resolution.

One method for increasing the spatial resolution of a small organ, such as the heart, is *zooming*. Zooming can be done at either the hardware or software levels. Figure 5-3A shows an image acquired onto a 6 x 6 matrix in the normal non-zoomed option. In the normal or non-zoomed mode, the amplification factor for the signals are calibrated such that the four edges of the 6 x 6 matrix are tangential to the circular field of view of the gamma camera. When acquiring an image in the *zoomed* mode (Fig. 5-3B), the signals for each count from the gamma camera are amplified by a factor greater than that used in the normal mode. In the case of software zoom, the coordinates of each scintillation event is multiplied by a predetermined zoom factor. As a result, counts from the central portion of the camera field of view are expanded to occupy the entire 6 x 6 matrix. Counts from the peripheral portion of the camera field of view are amplified out of the range of the image matrix and are lost from the display. Zooming is useful for decreasing the background counts and increasing the resolution through magnification when imaging a small organ such as the heart with a large field of view camera. Because some of the counts from the camera are discarded outside the array, the input count rate to the computer becomes lower. Also, there are a fewer number of counts per pixel in the resulting image for the same imaging time, so the noise of a zoomed image is increased. As previously explained, this problem can be solved by either increasing the imaging time in order to obtain the same number of counts or by increasing the dose to the patient to keep the acquisition time and the number of counts per image constant.

Of course, the spatial resolution of the computer image is ultimately limited by the resolution of the gamma camera. For a 40-cm diameter field of view gamma camera, the maximum camera resolution is adequately approximated by a 256 x 256 matrix. Given the current state of technology of gamma cameras, it would be a futile effort to gain resolution by acquiring data into a matrix larger than 256 x 256. If the acquisition matrix used is already 256 x 256, you would not gain spatial resolution by image zoom either, unless the purpose of the zoom was to eliminate counts from the

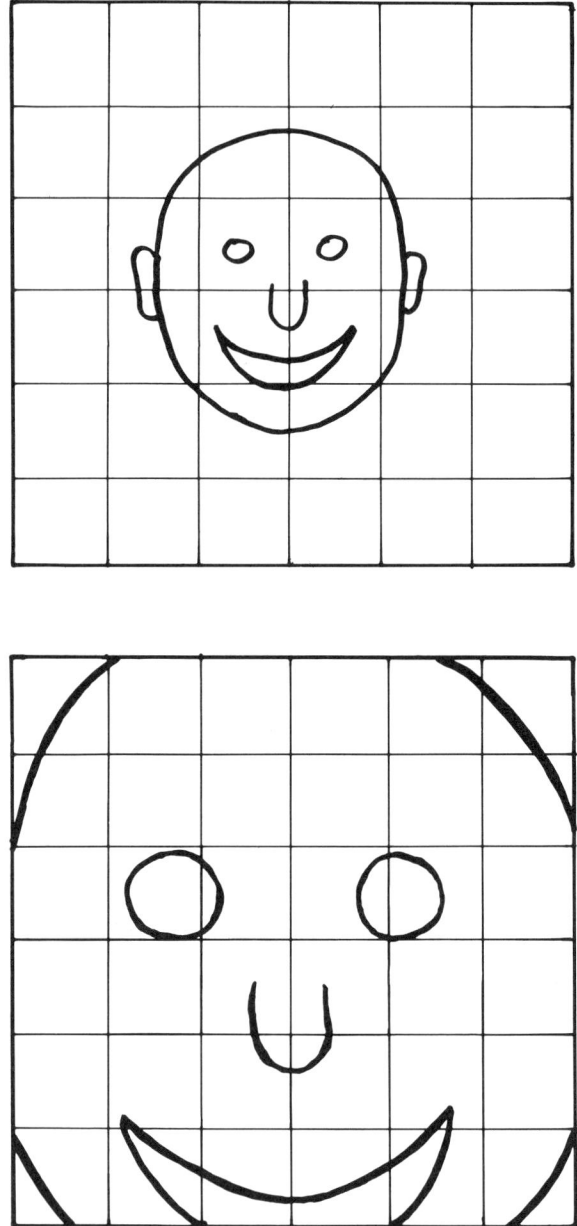

FIGURE 5-3 Zoom-mode acquisition magnifies the digitized image over many pixels to obtain the equivalent resolution of a larger image matrix.

undesired background. In this case, the image noise is reduced because most of the counts acquired to form the radionuclide image come from the organ of interest and not the background.

BYTE-MODE VERSUS WORD-MODE ACQUISITION

In the above discussion, a pixel was treated as though it could hold an unlimited number of counts. In reality the storage capacity of a pixel has a finite maximum. An image matrix has thus far been described as row and columns of storage elements called pixels. To fully describe the storage capacity of a pixel, we need to specify a third dimension, the depth of each pixel. In Figure 5-4, the depth of a pixel is determined by the number of bytes of computer memory used to form the pixel. In Figure 5-4A, one byte was used to form a pixel, while in Figure 5-4B two bytes were used. As you may recall, one byte consists of 8 bits, and two bytes form one word in a 16-bit computer, a common type of computer used in nuclear medicine. Therefore, a complete description of the image matrix must include the number of bytes used to form a pixel, in addition to the number of rows and columns of pixels in the matrix. Sometimes, the terms

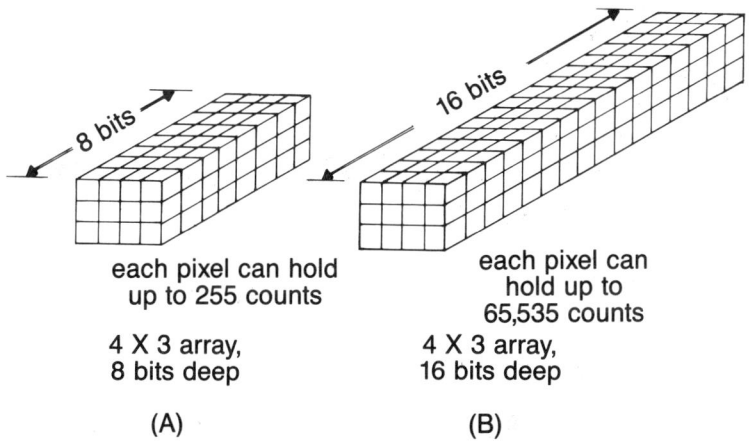

FIGURE 5-4 Word-mode acquisition (A) allows more counts to accumulate in each pixel than the byte mode in (B), but twice as much disk and memory space is required for each image.

byte-mode acquisition and *word-mode acquisition* are used to describe frame mode acquisition using a byte or a word to form one pixel, respectively.

When acquiring data into a pixel one-byte deep, the maximum number of counts that the pixel can hold is 255 ($2^8 - 1$). This is the largest number that eight bits can represent. If a pixel is given more than 255 counts, the extra counts will simply spill over and not be recorded into the computer memory. Whenever pixel saturation occurs, the image contrast and resolution are reduced because all the saturated pixels have exactly 255 counts. Quantitative analysis of the image over the saturated pixels also becomes impossible because count density changes in the region over the saturated pixels cannot be measured.

In using word-mode acquisition, each pixel is 16 bits deep; therefore the maximum number of counts that a 16-bit pixel can hold is ($2^{16} - 1$) or 65,535 counts. It is unlikely that a pixel will ever be filled with this many counts. Hence, pixel saturation will not occur in any foreseeable radionuclide image. Unfortunately, word-mode acquisition is wasteful because a large number of bits in the array will never be used, but it does not run the risk of count saturation as in the case of byte mode acquisition. For many low-count studies, such as brain flow and bone scans, byte-mode acquisition could certainly be used with little likelihood of encountering pixel saturation. For studies such as cardiac blood-pool and liver scans, pixel saturation will occur in critical areas of the anatomy when acquiring the data in the byte mode.

In the early days of nuclear medicine computers, computer memory and mass storage devices were expensive. Most radionuclide images were acquired in byte mode using 32 x 32 or 64 x 64 image matrices by necessity. Various data compression techniques had to be devised to protect a pixel from count overflow. One such technique is to allocate two or more byte arrays to hold the counts during acquisition. If during acquisition, any pixel in an array reached 255 counts before the acquisition time expires, all subsequent counts are shifted to the next array, and so on. Upon termination of the acquisition, counts in the corresponding pixels of all the arrays are added together in the central processing unit (CPU) and scaled to a value below 255. The scale factor along with the scaled pixel counts are then stored on the disk. The true number of counts in any pixel is recalled by multiplying the stored value by the scale factor.

One of the problems with scaled byte-mode acquisition is that there is a deadtime associated with shifting from one array to another; counts arriving during the deadtime are lost forever. For static acquisitions controlled by a preset number of counts, the deadtime prolongs the acquisition time by only an insignificant amount. However, for dynamic studies with high counting rates, the counts missed during the deadtime are valuable information lost from the study. Secondly, the counts for a pixel are stored and manipulated in the computer as integers, numbers without a fractional part. Truncation errors can be introduced during the scaling process. For example, if a pixel containing 17 counts is to be scaled by factor of 2, the stored value for that pixel is 8 instead of 8.5 (17/2 = 8.5) because the decimal part is truncated. Conversely, when the scaled value in storage for that pixel is converted back to obtain its true pixel count, the number becomes 16 instead of 17 because the decimal fraction was discarded during the scaling process.

Word-mode acquisition does not have truncation and deadtime problems but requires more computer memory and disk storage space. Now that computer memory and disk storage media are cheap and plentiful, the only reason for not acquiring images using 128 x 128 and 256 x 256 matrices in word mode, thus alleviating the problems of limited resolution and count overflow, is the concern for reduced count statistics in each pixel.

DYNAMIC FRAME-MODE ACQUISITION

With dynamic frame-mode acquisition, the computer is instructed to acquire a series of images, each for a predetermined length of time. This method of serial image acquisition is useful for the visualization and quantification of flow kinetics of a radionuclide. In the many years B.C. ("before computers"), flow studies such as the renogram were performed by recording onto Polaroid film an image of the radionuclide passing through the kidneys. One sheet of film was pulled every minute for 30 minutes. If a renogram is done on the computer using the dynamic frame acquisition method, the procedure is similar. Here, the computer takes over the responsibility of the technologist and the Polaroid camera for image recording and frame switching at the proper time intervals. Before acquisition begins, the operator enters into the computer the acquisition time for each frame, any time delay between frames, and the total number of frames to acquire in a given time interval. The number of frames that the computer is instructed to acquire per unit of time is called the framing rate. Once the acquisition is initiated, the technologist can relax and let the computer worry about collecting the counts into the CPU or buffer memory for each time interval.

For older computers with a limited amount of memory in the CPU or the frame buffer, the acquired image is emptied from the buffer memory to the disk at the end of each acquisition time period. The cycle is then repeated for the next image until the total number of frames or imaging time is reached. The problem with this type of computer is that when the CPU is transferring a set of image data to the disk, the computer is unresponsive to any new input data. Thus, the maximum framing rate the computer can handle is determined by the speed that an image matrix can be transferred or written onto the disk. This speed is dependent on a number of variables such as disk drive speed, data transfer rate of the disk, matrix size, and the number of users on-line, etc. The maximum framing rate stated in the user's manual is merely an approximation under typical conditions. The true maximum framing rate for a given computer installation will have to be determined at the user's site.

For these older computers, the framing rate can be increased by using a smaller image matrix, say using a 64 x 64 instead of a 128 x 128 matrix because the smaller matrix has a fewer number of bytes to transfer to the disk and thus reduces disk delays. However, in using a smaller matrix we are sacrificing spatial resolution (ability to see image details) for a higher temporal resolution (ability to separate the occurrence of events within a short time interval). For rapid dynamic studies, the chance for a pixel to acquire more than 255 counts in a short time interval is rather slim. Therefore, a pixel can be represented by one byte without fear of pixel saturation and shortage of disk storage space.

The newer computers with several megabytes or more of memory in the frame buffer can acquire and store a complete series of dynamic images without making room for the next image by transferring the previous images to the disk. Deadtime is greatly reduced when acquiring data on a computer with a large buffer memory.

Consequently, not only is a higher framing rate possible, but count statistics are also improved.

Frequently, we are not certain of the optimum framing rate to use for a special dynamic study. My suggestion is to use as high a framing rate as the computer can handle. Once the framing rate is determined, the temporal resolution will be only as high as the shortest time interval between two frames of images. We will not be able to obtain a finer temporal resolution by subdividing each image into two or more images of a shorter time interval because the arrival time of each count in an image frame is not recorded. A high framing rate gives good temporal resolution, but the statistical noise in the image may be high due to the limited number of counts collected in a short time interval. However, at the expense of reduced temporal resolution, two or more image frames can be added together to improve the spatial resolution.

MULTIPLE-GATED AND LIST-MODE ACQUISITION

Since multiple-gated and list-mode acquisitions are used almost exclusively with cardiac studies, detailed discussions on these two acquisition methods will be addressed in Chapter 8. It will suffice to say that multiple-gated acquisition is a special type of dynamic-frame acquisition that uses a physiologic signal, such as the patient's ECG pulse, to synchronize the framing rate and the framing sequence.

Although multiple-gated acquisition is almost synonymous with dynamic heart studies, it has been used with a small degree of success for synchronizing acquisition of lung images with respiration motion.

The list mode was necessary with the older, slower computers for short duration acquisition at very high transient count rates. Cardiac first-pass studies are good examples of short duration, rapid dynamic acquisitions because they involve collecting counts in excess of 50,000 cps over a 30-second period. With the advent of high-speed computers, disk drives, and abundant memory, the use of list mode for the acquisition of radionuclide images has virtually disappeared.

CONCLUSION

Discussions on radionuclide image processing tend to concentrate on the various methods of manipulating the data to improve the appearance of the image or extracting quantitative information from the data. However, we must keep in mind the law of "Conservation of Ignorance," which reminds us that we cannot get any information that was never present in the data. This law is quite applicable to radionuclide image processing. Unless the necessary data have been acquired into the computer, all the exotic image processing techniques ever developed by man will never give us the desired information. Hopefully, a better understanding of the various steps involved in the acquisition of radionuclide images into the computer may help the reader to avoid many of the pitfalls that could spoil the entire patient study.

SUGGESTED READINGS

1. Cradduck TD. Computers in nuclear medicine. *Radiographics* 1985;5:51-81.
2. Erickson JJ. Nuclear medicine computers—software. *J Nucl Med Technol* 1985;13:97-105.
3. Erickson JJ. Nuclear medicine computer systems—hardware. *J Nucl Med Technol* 1985;13:140-161.
4. King MA, Zimmerman RE, Links JM. *Imaging hardware and software for nuclear medicine.* New York: American Association of Physicists in Medicine; 1988.
5. Gelfano MJ, Thomas SR. *Effective use of computers in nuclear medicine: practical clinical applications in the imaging laboratory.* New York: MacGraw-Hill; 1988.
6. Liberman DE. *Computer methods—the fundamentals of digital nuclear medicine.* St. Louis: CV Mosby; 1977.

CHAPTER

6

METHODS OF QUALITATIVE IMAGE ANALYSIS

INTRODUCTION

Data acquisition programs constitute only a small fraction of the clinical software package available with each nuclear medicine computer system. The majority of clinical software packages consist of programs that can be classified under one of the following three general categories: (1) image enhancement, (2) quantitative analysis, and (3) image reconstruction for emission computed tomography. At some institutions, the nuclear medicine computer also is being used for report generation and departmental recordkeeping. In this chapter, we will discuss some of the common methods of digital image processing techniques for enhancing the appearance of radionuclide images.

IMAGE ENHANCEMENT

Image enhancement is the process of utilizing a computer to transform an image from one form of presentation to another in order to bring out the desired features on the display. In the early days of image processing, the computer was used merely as an image storage device. Using the count data stored in the computer, repeat exposures were made on photographic film by trial and error until the proper film density was obtained, thus saving much time from having to do repeat scanning of the patient. This same task can be handled by many analog devices, but they do not offer the flexibility of a digital computer.

Since this modest beginning, image processing software has expanded to include sophisticated algorithms to: (1) enhance specific features in the original image, (2) manipulate the presentation of the image, (3) correct for distortions caused by image acquisition devices, and (4) perform other mathematical analyses to extract diagnostic information for patient management. This large variety of operations is made possible by having the image data stored in the computer in numerical form, which allows it to be manipulated mathematically.

CONVOLUTION METHODS OF IMAGE ENHANCEMENT

Image Smoothing Filters

One of the earliest attempts to improve the quality of radionuclide images employed smoothing filters to reduce image noise. For now, let us define image noise as undesired and distracting details blended in with the radionuclide image due to the relatively few number of counts collected for each image. As a result of noise interference, a solid surface appears fuzzy and the edges show up jagged. A common method used for improving the quality of the radionuclide image is to remove the unwanted noise by passing a smoothing filter through the input image. A smoothing filter is a fancy name for a way of suppressing the noise by averaging the pixel counts in the image. The familiar nine-point smoothing filter is one such example of a pixel averaging method. The nine-point smooth procedure illustrated in Figure 6-1 uses a 4 x 4 image matrix. For a given pixel in the image array, say P7, the number of counts in that pixel (20 in this example) is replaced by a new value equal to the average of the surrounding pixels. The simplest way of calculating the new pixel value for P7 is by adding together the number of counts in pixel P7 and the counts in each of the eight surrounding pixels, and then dividing the sum by nine:

$$\text{Avg} = (P_2 + P_3 + P_4 + P_6 + P_7 + P_8 + P_{10} + P_{11} + P_{12})/9$$
$$\text{Avg} = (30 + 40 + 150 + 70 + 20 + 100 + 10 + 90 + 50)/9$$
$$= 62.2$$

QUALITATIVE IMAGE ANALYSIS   101

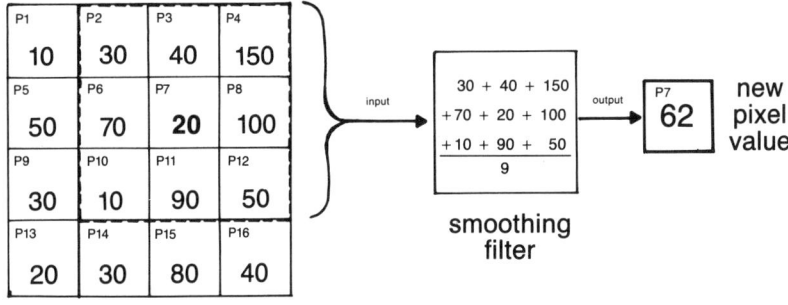

FIGURE 6-1 The simple average filter changes the counts in the center pixel (P7) to the average of the nine pixels within the mask.

As a result of the above calculation, the number of counts in pixel P7 is changed from 20 to 62, after dropping the fraction. To smooth the entire image array, the same algorithm is applied to pixels P6, P10, and P11. The result from each calculation is saved in another image array and plotted (see Fig. 6-2). Notice that the counts in pixels lying along the edge of the matrix (i.e., P1, P2, P3, P4, P5, P8, P9, P12, P13, P14, P15, P16) are not replaced because some

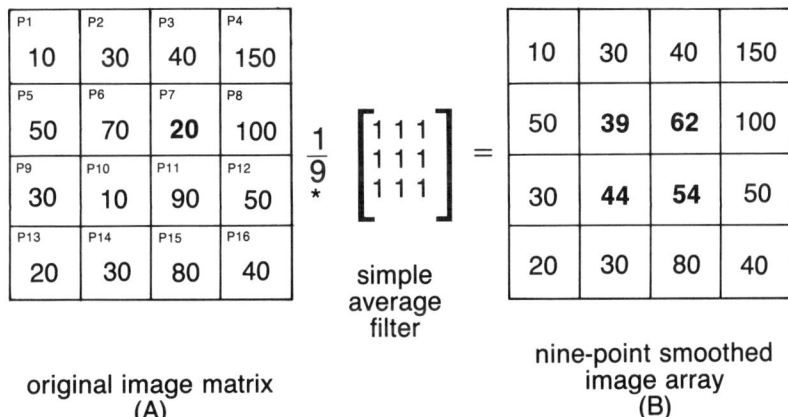

FIGURE 6-2 A simple nine-point smoothed image is obtained by moving the mask over the image matrix. At each stop, it replaces the value in the center pixel by the average of the nine pixel counts within the mask.

of their surrounding pixels lie outside the matrix, and thus become unavailable for averaging. Review the calculation in Figure 6-1 for at least another pixel to see how Figure 6-2 was produced.

In effect, the nine-point smoothing involves moving a mask over the entire radionuclide image. This mask consists of 3 x 3 block of pixels, each having a value equal to 1/9. As the mask is superimposed over a block of nine pixels in the input radionuclide image, it makes the center pixel look more like its neighbors by replacing the original pixel count with the average of the counts for the nine pixels. As this mask continues to move over the entire input image, each of the center pixels becomes more like its surrounding neighbors. At the end of its journey, a blurred output image is created, due to the mask (or convolution kernel) making each pixel less distinguishable from its neighbors. The process of smearing an input radionuclide image with a blurring pixel mask can be equivalently expressed as performing a *convolution filter* on the input image using a smoothing kernel.

The nine-point smoothing filter in Figure 6-1 assumes that each of the neighborhood pixels affects the counts in the center pixel equally. More generally, a smoothing convolution kernel assumes that a pixel lying farther away from the center gives lesser influence than the ones located centrally. A widely used nine-point smoothing filter weights the 3 x 3 block of pixels as follows:

$$\frac{1}{16}\begin{bmatrix} 1 & 2 & 1 \\ 2 & 4 & 2 \\ 1 & 2 & 1 \end{bmatrix}$$

meaning that counts in the center pixel should be given the most important consideration during averaging, and thus are weighted twice as much as the counts in the immediate neighborhood pixels. Being farthest away from the center pixel, counts in pixels lying in the diagonal corners of the mask are considered the least important; hence, they are weighted only one-fourth as much during pixel averaging. In calculating the average of the center pixel:

$$P_7 = \frac{1}{16}\begin{bmatrix} 1*P_2 + 2*P_3 + 1*P_4 + \\ 2*P_6 + 4*P_7 + 2*P_8 + \\ 1*P_{10} + 2*P_{11} + 1*P_{12} \end{bmatrix}$$

QUALITATIVE IMAGE ANALYSIS

or

$$P_7 = \frac{1}{16}\begin{bmatrix} 1*30 + 2*40 + 1*150 + \\ 2*70 + 4*20 + 2*100 + \\ 1*10 + 2*90 + 1*50 \end{bmatrix}$$

$$= 1/16 \, (920)$$

$$= 57.5$$

$$= 57 \text{ (dropping the fraction).}$$

The sum is divided by 16 because the total weight in the filter adds up to 16.

The above calculation shows that the weighted pixel average (57) is lower than the unweighted average (62) for P7. The weighted pixel averaging algorithm brings the counts in the center pixel closer to that of its neighbors, but not as much as in the case of unweighted pixel averaging. The output image therefore is less blurred and has a higher spatial resolution because the center pixel retains more of its original characteristics. The matrix in Figure 6-3 is the

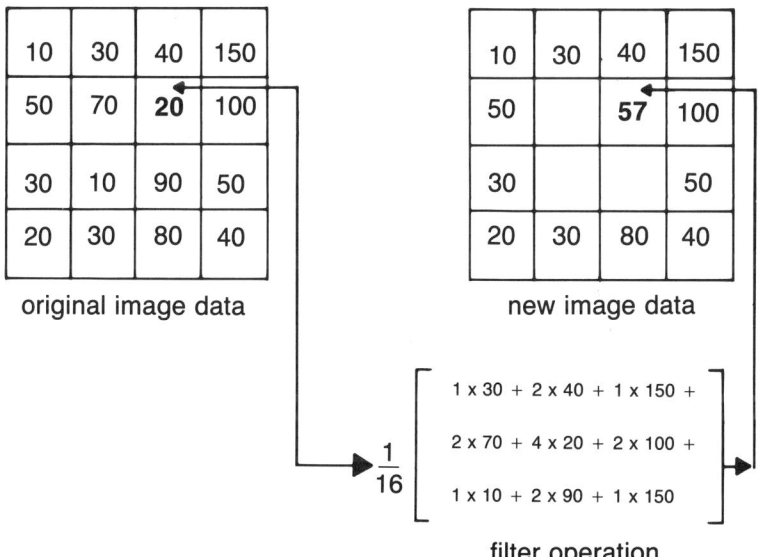

FIGURE 6-3 The number of counts in the center pixel is replaced by the weighted average of the nine pixels under the mask.

result of applying the weighted nine-point smoothing operation on the 5 x 5 image array in Figure 6-1.

In summary, the image smoothing procedure involves modifying the count distribution in the input image by moving a mask through each pixel in the original image. This pixel mask or convolution kernel, which is made up of an array of coefficients or modifying factors, is used to calculate a new value for a given pixel by taking a weighted average of the counts for each pixel under the mask. After multiplying the counts in each pixel under the mask with the corresponding weighting coefficient, the products are then added together to produce a weighted average for the center pixel. The general procedure for a 3 x 3 pixel convolution is illustrated in Figure 6-4. The lower case letters, **a, b, c, d, e, f, g, h, i,** are the weights or coefficients in the 3 x 3 convolution kernel, while the upper case letters **A, B, C, D, E, F, G, H, I,** are the corresponding pixel counts in the input image, with E^1 being the smoothed value. If all the weights in the mask are equal, the output pixel count is just a simple average of its neighborhood pixel counts. Otherwise, the output image pixel is a weighted pixel average.

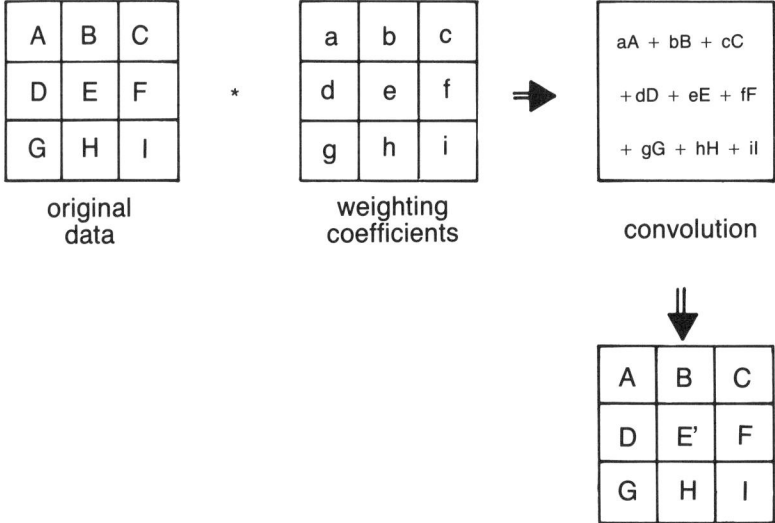

FIGURE 6-4 The procedure for convolution of the original image matrix with the filter kernel to produce the processed image matrix.

The new pixel average does not, however, replace the original pixel value in the input image. Instead, a separate matrix is created to store the new pixel averages and to form a new output image. If the new pixel average replaces the original pixel value in the input image, you will gradually distort the pixel averages to be calculated later. Distortion is produced because the pixel you just changed in the input image is a neighborhood pixel for the next pixel you are about to change. As the pixel mask moves over the entire input image, the neighborhood pixels deviate more and more from their original values.

Using the pixel averaging or convolution filter as an image smoothing algorithm can be described as *replace averaging*. The basic idea is to produce a new image by substituting the original pixel count with one modified by the mask. Many diverse effects on the original image can be produced by assigning different weighting factors in the pixel mask and by using different sizes of pixel masks. Median image smoothing and edge detection are examples of image manipulation by varying the coefficients in the convolution kernel.

Median smoothing is a type of replace averaging in that the value of the center pixel is replaced by the median pixel instead of the weighted average of the pixel counts in the mask. The median pixel is the pixel whose count value is greater than 50% of the pixels in the mask, but is also lower than 50% of the pixels. The number of counts in the median pixel is exactly at the half-way mark. The median filter is useful for eliminating contribution from pixels containing extreme values.

Edge-Enhancement Filters

Edge enhancement is an opposite operation to image smoothing. While image smoothing attempts to reduce the contrast between adjacent pixels, edge enhancement aims to accentuate the contrast between two adjacent pixels. Interestingly, edge enhancement can be carried out using the same pixel replace averaging technique used for image smoothing. The only difference lies in the coefficients that make up the pixel mask. If the center pixel of the mask is given a positive weight and the surrounding pixels are negative, then convolution of the input image with the *sharpening mask* yields a new image that emphasizes the edges and sharp details. An example of edge enhancement using the convolution or replace pixel averaging technique is shown in Figure 6-5.

The pixel mask always carries an odd number of rows and columns of pixels so that there is always a pixel in the exact center of the mask. The dimensions of the mask, measured in terms of the number of pixels along each side of the array, varies according to the equation:

$$(2N + 1) \times (2N + 1).$$

If $N = 1$, the mask is 3 x 3; if $N = 2$, the mask is 5 x 5, and so on. In general, a large pixel mask will do a better job in removing the unwanted noise without oversmoothing the original image. However, the time required for convolution with a large pixel mask may be so long that it may be impractical in a clinical environment. As you can see, whenever the dimension of the mask is doubled, there is a four-fold increase in the number of pixels in the mask, hence a four-fold increase in the computation time. Time-saving is the principal reason why the 3 x 3 pixel mask is so widely used.

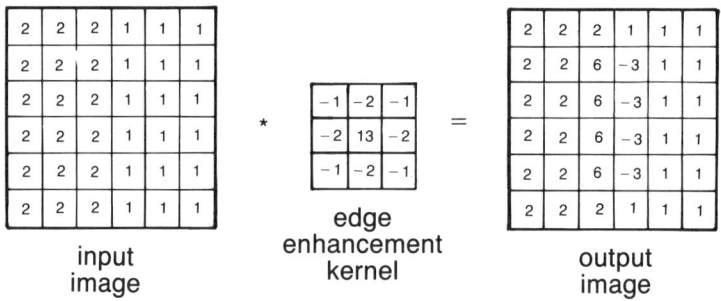

FIGURE 6-5 The edge contrast is increased from 2:1 to 9:1 after taking a convolution of the original image with an edge-enhancement filter. Edge-enhancement filters typically place positive coefficients in the center and negative in the periphery.

FOURIER METHODS OF IMAGE ENHANCEMENT

Convolution filters manipulate data in the space domaine, i.e., points, lines and intensity variables. An alternate method to the convolution filtering for image smoothing or edge enhancement is to use a Fourier filter. The end result of a Fourier filter is the same as that of a convolution filter, except that the Fourier filter manipulates the image data in the frequency domain instead of the space domain. In fact, the Fourier filter is an exact mathematical equivalence of a convolution filter.

Fundamentals of Fourier Analysis

When working with a Fourier filter, the image data are represented as a series of sine and cosine waves, each with a different spatial frequency, phase and amplitude. Image smoothing or edge enhancement is achieved by eliminating or suppressing the high and low frequency component waves, respectively, which is why a Fourier filter is also known as a spatial frequency filter. An intuitive approach to understanding Fourier filtering is as follows. The process of removing the unwanted frequencies in an image involves three distinct steps: (1) transforming the image from the space domain into the frequency domain; (2) selectively attenuating the amplitude of the undesired frequencies; and (3) transforming the modified image in the frequency domain back to the space domain.

The major stumbling block to the understanding of Fourier filters lies in that first step: transforming the image into the frequency domain. How can we transform a visual image from the world of points, lines and planes along with their colors or shades of gray to the mystical world of frequency and amplitude? The metamorphosis is easy to understand if we just think about the relationship between the music written by the composer and the music played by the orchestra.

The orchestra produces a composite sound that changes from one moment to the next as the different instruments play their own tunes with different loudness and at different time sequences. The music can be saved for posterity by using a tape recorder to record the moment-by-moment variations of the air pressure against the microphone. The method that records the sound as a function of time is said to operate in the time domain.

On the other hand, an aspiring music composer could transcribe the sound of the orchestra to a set of notes on a music scale. You may not think of it in this fashion, but each note on a music scale actually represents a unique sound frequency. In addition to the notes on a scale, a music score also describes the precise moment that a note should begin and the relative loudness that note should be played, i.e., the phase and amplitude of each note. Thus, a music score describes each note to be played by the instruments in terms of the frequency, amplitude, and phase of the sound. The method that records a sound in terms of the phase and amplitude of its various frequencies is said to work in the frequency domain. In so doing, the aspiring music composer is doing a Fourier transform of the music played by the orchestra from the time domain to the frequency domain. When a musician reads the music score and produces a sound using his instrument, he is doing an *inverse Fourier transform*. Here, the music is changed from the frequency domain to the time domain. Basically, Fourier transform is just a way to transcribe information from one set of notations to another.

Although a time-varying function was used as an example, Fourier analysis can be used to solve a variety of problems involving mathematical functions that can be approximated by a sum of periodic waves. In nuclear medicine, we utilize the Fourier method to describe the resolution of a gamma camera and to manipulate information stored in a radionuclide image. Likewise, in many image analysis situations, it is easier to first transform the image to the frequency domain, work it over to eliminate the noise and other undesired frequencies, and then transform it back to the spatial domain. The extra work in transforming the image back and forth between the space and frequency domains is well worth it, considering the flexibility of the Fourier method in performing a wide variety of operations.

Fourier Image Filters

Keeping the analogy of describing music in the frequency domain, let us apply the same methodology to image analysis. Fourier analysis makes the assumption that a mathematical function can be represented by a sum of sine and cosine waves of different frequency, amplitude, and phase. Figure 6-6 shows that we can reconstruct a square wave with two sharp corners by adding together a series of sine waves. As more high frequency terms are added to the sum, the corner becomes sharper and sharper. This simple geometric figure illustrates one important concept in the analysis of any image in the frequency domain. A large number of high frequency terms is required to describe the sharp corners, while only a few low frequency, slowly varying waves are sufficient to build up the flat-topped section of the square wave. In other words, the fine details and sharp edges of an image are predominantly made up of high frequency waves, while the low resolution portion of an image contains mostly low frequency wave components.

Now let us go one step deeper into transforming a radionuclide image from the space domain to the frequency domain. Since the data for a radionuclide image are stored in the computer in numerical form, it can be translated to a set of mathematical functions.

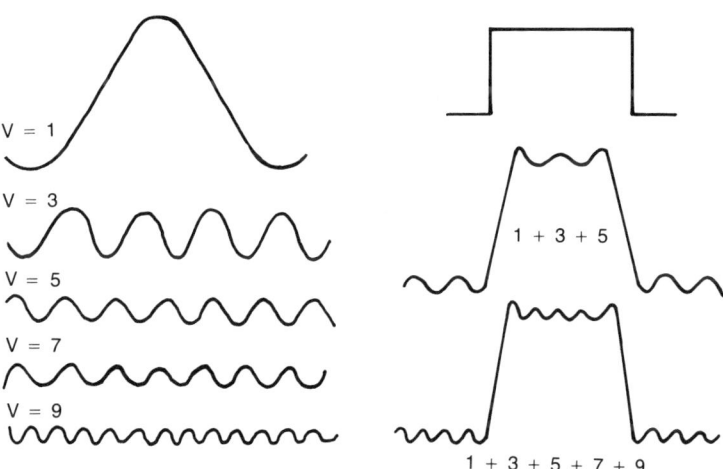

FIGURE 6-6 A square wave can be constructed from a sum of sine waves. Compared to low-frequency waves, high-frequency waves have lower amplitudes and contribute less to the overall strength of the square wave. However, they are needed to render the appearance of a square wave, especially the sharp corners.

Our ulterior motive is to transform this set of mathematical functions to the frequency domain by Fourier transform. The idea that a body organ, such as the liver, can be described by a set of mathematical equations is not so ridiculous after analyzing an ordinary image such as the liver and spleen scan in Figure 6-7.

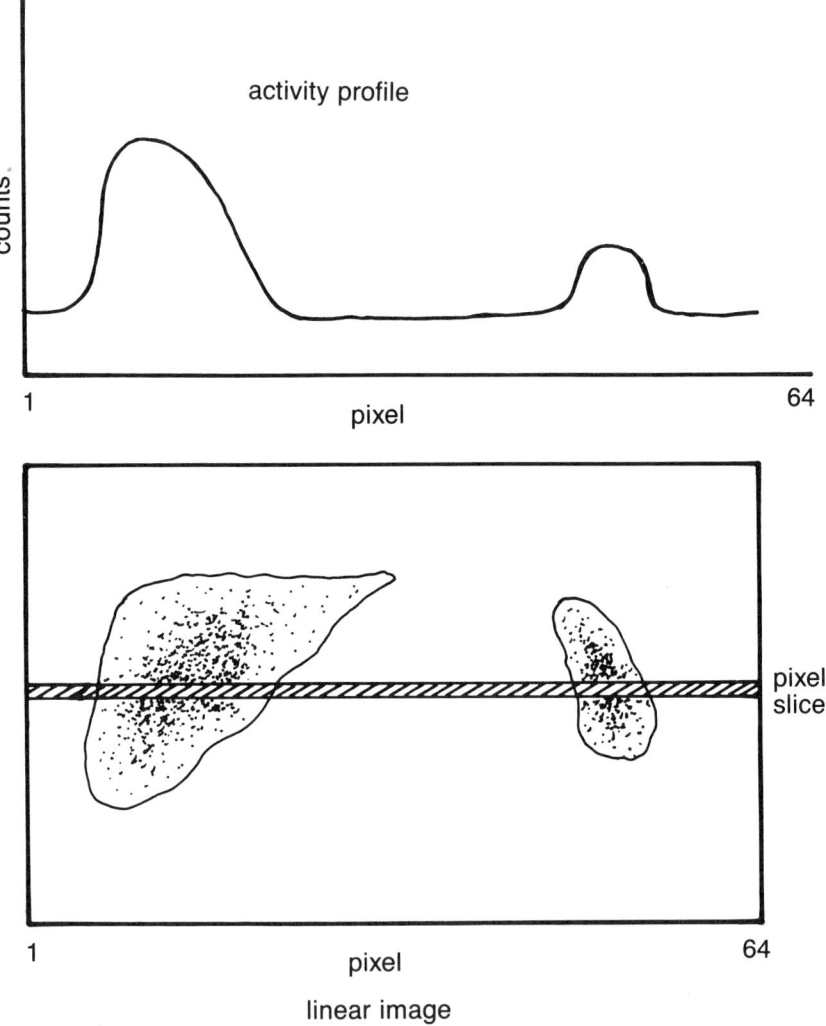

FIGURE 6-7 An activity profile is a plot of the counts in pixels lying along a line. The activity profile in this example is a plot of the counts along a horizontal row of pixels.

Assume this scan was acquired in a 64 x 64 matrix. If we plot on a graph the number of counts in each pixel across one row of the matrix, say the 34th row, we obtain a curve with 64 data points as in Figure 6-7. In nuclear medicine jargon, we call such a curve an activity profile. For a 64 x 64 matrix, we can do the same for each row of pixels and obtain a set of 64 activity profiles. However, a curve plot is actually a graphic representation of a mathematical function. Hence, an activity profile is a graphic representation of a mathematical function. In a 64 x 64 image matrix there would be 64 equations, and a 128 x 128 image matrix is actually made up of 128 simultaneous equations.

Using the Fourier transform, the equation representing the activity profile in Figure 6-7 is reconstructed as a sum of a number of sine and cosine terms, each with a different amplitude and frequency. The mathematical operations involved with Fourier transform are described in Appendix C. We only need to note that Fourier transform is just a mathematical recipe for the computer to crank out the phase and amplitude (also known as the Fourier coefficients) of all the frequencies that make up the activity profile. After performing a Fourier transform on each row of pixels in the image matrix, we have accomplished moving the image data from the space domain to the frequency domain.

The next task is to filter out the unwanted frequencies from the image. Recall from the description of the frequency components in the square wave of Figure 6-6 that the high-frequency terms are responsible for the sharp edges and fine details. Unfortunately, these high-frequency terms become imbedded with a large amount of statistical noise. The edges of an organ often give a fuzzy appearance because they are predominantly made up of high frequency components and these components contain a high statistical noise due to the relatively few number of counts collected in the region. These distracting high frequency components can be suppressed using a low-pass filter, also known as a smoothing filter. A low-pass filter acts like a sieve, permitting only those components with a low frequency to pass through and eliminating those components with a high frequency. As a result, the filtered image looks more pleasing with a smooth display, but the details are blurred because the high-frequency components are attenuated by the smoothing filter. If the square wave in Figure 6-6 is operated on by a low-pass filter, the high frequencies will be removed in the process, and the resultant image will have a rounded corner instead of a sharp 90° turn.

The low-pass filtering process is performed by multiplying the amplitudes of the high-frequency components in the original image by a modifying factor having a value between 0 and 1. If the amplitude of a frequency is multiplied by 0, contribution from that frequency to the resulting image is eliminated. Expression of that frequency in the output image display is de-emphasized if the multiplication factor is greater than 0 but greater than 1.

Image manipulation in the frequency domain is just as flexible as the convolution method in the space domain. If we want to enhance the edges, we would use a high-pass filter to let all the high-frequency components pass through and eliminate or suppress the low-frequency components in the output image.

If we desire the ouput image to contain only those features within a limited range of frequencies, we would use a band-pass filter. A band-pass filter is a mathematical sieve that permits only those terms within a limited band of frequencies to pass through and eliminates all other components with frequencies above or below the permissible band of frequencies. The function of a band-pass filter is thus identical to that of the pulse-height analyzer in the gamma camera, which permits only those photon pulses within a certain window of energy to pass.

The final step in the Fourier filtering process is to bring the modified image data from the frequency domain back to the space domain. The mathematical procedure for this final step, inverse Fourier transform, is discussed in Appendix C. Please note that only one technique utilizing one-dimensional Fourier transform has been discussed. Many Fourier image processing techniques, however, utilize a two-dimensional Fourier transform. Contrary to what you have heard before, two-dimensional Fourier transform is not an incomprehensible mathematical procedure. To do a two-dimensional Fourier transform, simply apply a one-dimensional Fourier transform twice. First do a one-dimensional Fourier transform for each row of pixels as previously described. Then do a one-dimensional transform again on each resulting column of Fourier coefficients. That is all there is to two-dimensional Fourier transform.

Both the Fourier and convolution filters can do the same job in removing the undesired features from the input radionuclide image. However, the convolution technique is more often used than the Fourier method for nuclear medicine image processing. One of the reasons is the computation time. The convolution technique is faster than the Fourier technique when the kernels are smaller than 9 x 9. Since most nuclear medicine images can be adequately processed using a 3 x 3 kernel, the Fourier technique is not often used. However, with the advent of high speed computers or the aid of a special hardware device, the array processor which can perform Fourier transform in a fraction of the time it used to take, time is no longer the prime consideration. More importantly, serious ring artifacts can be generated and propagated throughout the image if we are careless with the computation details of Fourier transform, which is one of the prime reasons why the convolution technique is preferred for most image smoothing or edge-enhancement operations.

POINT PROCESSING OPERATIONS

Although the convolution and the Fourier filters share the spot light in every discussion of computer image processing, the simple point arithmetic operations are just as important. Contrary to the convolution and Fourier techniques in which the number of counts in a pixel is modified according to the counts in the surrounding pixels, the point processing techniques manipulate the number of counts in a pixel that can be completely independent of its neighbors.

Background Subtraction

One example of a neighborhood-independent points processing operation is contrast enhancement whereby a constant number of counts is subtracted from each pixel in the image. This pixel-by-pixel count subtraction operation, commonly referred to as background subtraction, is routinely used to improve the contrast of radionuclide images. Figure 6-8A shows a hot spot with 200 counts/pixel against a background of 100 counts/pixel. The target-to-non-target ratio is

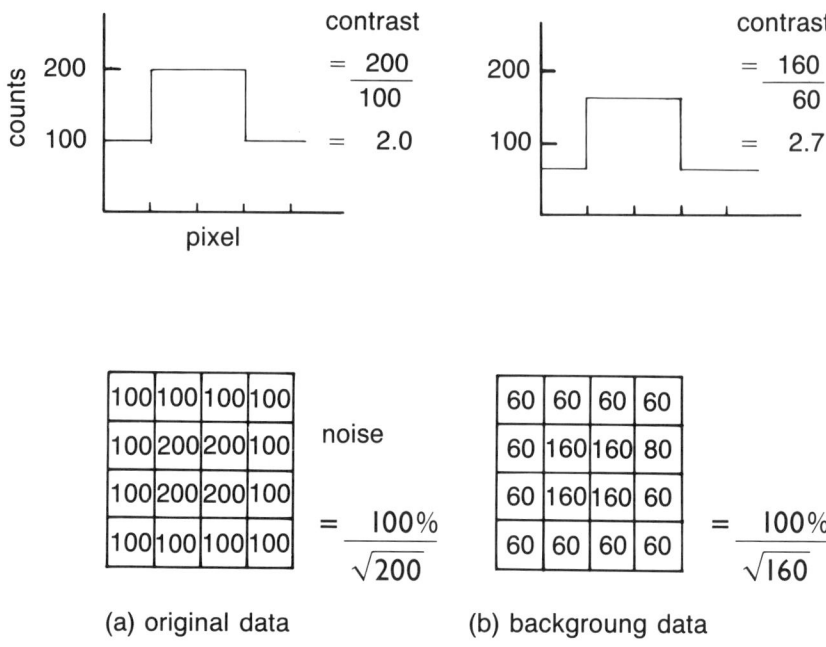

FIGURE 6-8 The simple background subtraction method subtracts a constant number of counts from each pixel to increase the target-to-background ratio.

2:1. If we subtract 20% of the counts in the hot spot (i.e., 40 counts) from every pixel in the image, we get the image shown in Figure 6-8B. As a result of subtracting 40 counts from every pixel in the image, the target and background counts become 160 and 60 counts/pixel, respectively, and the contrast is increased from 2:1 to 2.7:1.

One may argue that the number of counts to be subtracted as background is largely decided on the basis of the average pixel counts in the surrounding pixels. However, the fact remains that the number of counts to be subtracted was determined before the operation began and that the same number of counts was subtracted from every pixel regardless of the neighborhood that the pixel happened to be in. Thus, this point processing operation is a pure pixel-by-pixel translation according to a predetermined function.

Interpolated Background Subtraction

Interpolated background subtraction is a neighborhood-dependent point operation and is usually applied to enhance the target-background ratio of ^{201}Tl myocardial perfusion images. Unlike the simple background subtraction, which assumes an uniform background activity, the interpolated background subtraction technique assumes that the amount of background activity in the radionuclide image varies, depending upon the neighborhood. The appropriate number of counts to be subtracted from a given pixel should, by interpolation, reflect the quantity of activity in the surrounding background pixels. The interpolation is carried out by calculating a weighted average of the activity of its immediate background pixels.

Using the interpolated background subtraction method, the myocardial image is first bracketed inside a rectangle (Fig. 6-9). All

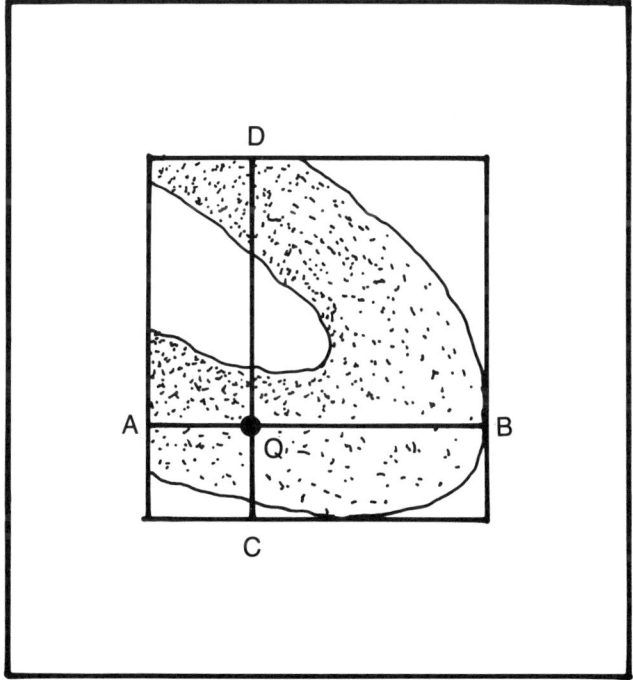

FIGURE 6-9 The interpolated background subtraction method subtracts from each pixel a number equal to the weighted average of the counts in four pixels at the edge of the ROI.

pixels outside the rectangle are considered the background. The immediate background pixels are those pixels lying along the boundaries of the rectangle.

Suppose we want to subtract the background activity from the pixel labeled Q inside the rectangle. The background activities of its four immediate background pixels are labeled A, B, C, and D; those background pixels are located at a distance of X_a, X_b, Y_c and Y_d, respectively, from Q. The background activity, Bkg, to be subtracted from point Q is calculated as the weighted average of the activity located at points A, B, C and D as follows:

$$Bkg = \frac{W_a A + W_b B + W_c C + W_d D}{W_a + W_b + W_c + W_d}$$

There are several ways to assign weights to the activity for each background pixel. One method is to assign weights to each of the background pixels equally:

$$W_a = W_b = W_c = W_d = 1$$

The background to be subtracted from Q is simply the average of the counts in the four surrounding boundary pixels.

More commonly, the weight assigned to each background pixel is a different value. The distance-weighted average assumes that the background activity in pixel Q is more strongly influenced by the nearby background pixels than those lying farther away. The weight assigned to each of the background pixels is calculated as follows:

$$W_a = X_b / X_a$$

$$W_b = X_a / X_b$$

$$W_c = Y_d / Y_c$$

$$W_d = Y_c / Y_d$$

Thus, the activity in a given background pixel is weighted inversely with its distance from Q. Both the weighted and unweighted interpolated background subtraction methods are neighborhood-dependent point processing operations. The activity to be subtracted varies from pixel to pixel within the rectangle, depending on the activities found in the perpendicular boundary pixels.

Gray Scales For Video Image Display

The gray level assignment for a pixel to be displayed on a black-and-white video monitor is an example of neighborhood-independent point processing. The assignment of a shade of gray to each pixel in an image is nothing more than translating the number of counts in a pixel to an integer which in turn defines the brightness that the pixel will appear on the video monitor. Usually the brightness of a pixel in a black-and-white monitor varies from completely black to completely white. The number of shades of gray between these two extremes is called the gray scale, or dynamic range. In most nuclear medicine computers, the gray scale consists of 256 shades of gray. Although scaling the image pixels to 256 levels of gray gives an aesthetically pleasing display with a continuous gray tone, this large number of gray levels is actually superfluous because the human eye can differentiate less than 128 shades of gray under ideal conditions. In fact, 64 gray levels are probably adequate for the display of most images.

The simplest form of gray scale transformation is the *linear gray scale,* which assigns a gray level directly proportional to the number of counts in the pixel. Using the 256-level gray scale given by Curve A in Figure 6-10 as an example, the pixel with the highest number of counts in the image matrix is white and the pixel with zero counts is black; all other pixels with counts between these two limits are assigned a gray level proportional to the ratio of the counts in the pixel to the maximum pixel count. The assignment of a gray level to each pixel is handled by a look-up table in the computer in which the pixel count is used as the input, and an integer is provided as the output to define how bright the pixel should be displayed on the monitor. The range of integers from 0 to 255 then defines the 256-step dynamic range of the gray scale.

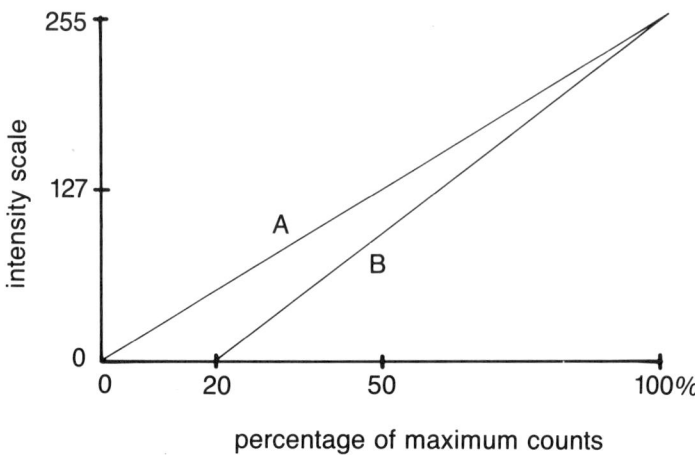

FIGURE 6-10 Both gray scales A and B normalize the display intensity to the maximum pixel counts. Scale B has a steeper slope than Scale A and gives a higher image contrast because the density scale is spread only over 80% of the counts.

Suppose that the highest pixel count in a 64 x 64 matrix is 480 counts. This pixel is assigned by the look-up table to level 255, the maximum pixel brightness. If a pixel has 240 counts, half the number of counts in the hottest pixel, its gray level is assigned 128. For a pixel with 120 counts, one-fourth of the maximum pixel counts, its gray level is 64, and so on.

Suppose in another image, the maximum number of counts in a pixel is 200, then the pixel with 200 counts would be assigned the maximum brightness level of 255. A pixel with 128 counts is assigned to the gray level of 163 (255 x 128/200), and a pixel with 64 counts is assigned to the gray level of 82 (255 x 64/200).

This method of gray level assignment is said to normalize pixel counts to the highest level in the gray scale, i.e., the hottest pixel is given the highest intensity on the display, and other pixels are shaded proportionately lower. Gray scale normalization makes full use of the entire gray scale and should be used for images with high count stati..ics. However, for images with poor count statistics such as where the maximum pixel count is only 100, normalizing the pixel counts to the maximum brightness can create sharp distinct bands of gray in the image. This distracting appearance is due to pixels being assigned to greatly varied gray levels for having only a slight difference in counts.

For images with poor count statistics, non-normalized gray scale assignment makes the image appear with more continuous shades of gray by using the non-normalized gray scale technique when the hottest pixel in an image is 200 counts, its gray level becomes 200, while the pixels with 128 and 64 counts are assigned to the gray levels 128 and 64, respectively. With this method of gray level assignment, the dynamic range is limited, but the resulting image does not contain distracting bands of gray. The obvious problem with non-normalized gray level assignment for images with high count density is that it will saturate the pixel brightness in regions where the pixel counts exceed 255; all these pixels will appear completely white on the display no matter what the actual pixel counts are.

A variation of the linear gray scale is shown by Curve B in Figure 6-10. The gray scale renders any pixel with counts less than 20% of the maximum completely black on the display; the gray scale is occupied only by those pixels with counts between 20% to 100% of the maximum pixel count. This method of scaling the pixel brightness actually performs a background subtraction by eliminating from the display those pixels with counts less than the count threshold. Since Curve B has a steeper density gradient than Curve A, an image scaled according to Curve B will yield a higher contrast than if it was scaled according to Curve A and eliminating from the video display all the pixels with counts less than 20% of the maximum. Background subtraction by imposing a threshold on the gray scale is convenient because the operator can easily adjust the background threshold until the desired contrast is obtained. It must be emphasized, however, that imposing a threshold on the gray scale only eliminates the pixels with low counts from the video display. The number of counts stored in each pixel in the image matrix remains unchanged. On the other hand, the point-by-point background subtraction actually reduces the number of counts in each pixel.

The disadvantage of imposing a threshold on the gray scale is that information in the low count rate region is eliminated from the display. The gray scale as shown in Figure 6-11 changes the pixel density continuously as an exponential function of the counts. Such a non-linear gray scale gives a small density difference between pixels in the low count region and a large difference in the hot region. The exponential gray scale does not eliminate pixels in the low count region from the display. Instead, the exponential scale simply suppresses the contrast between pixels in the low count region and exaggerates the density of those in the high count region. This scheme is useful for increasing the contrast of pixels in the hot or high count region without eliminating from the display data in the low count region.

The gray scale given by Curve B in Figure 6-11 gives a logarithmic change in the displayed density as a function of the pixel counts. The logarithmic gray scale gives an opposite effect to that of the thresholding and exponential gray scales, in that the count difference between pixels in the low count region is emphasized, while the count difference between pixels in the high count region is suppressed. The logarithmic gray scale is useful for bringing out the contrast of pixels in the low count region. Unfortunately, some images when displayed with the logarithmic gray scale may show exaggerated distinct bands of gray in the low count regions that may be quite annoying to the viewer.

Exponential and logarithmic gray scales are used only occasionally because the artifical exaggeration and suppression of density

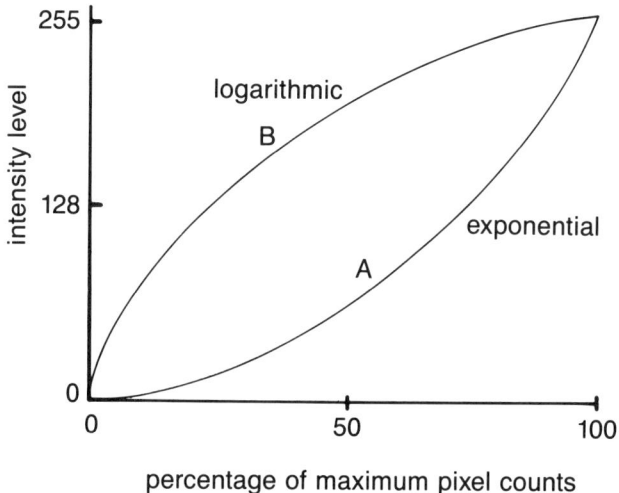

FIGURE 6-11 The logarithmic scale enhances image contrast in the low count region and suppresses the contrast in the high count region. The exponential scale give just the opposite effect.

differences between pixels may give a false impression of abnormal radionuclide distribution.

Color Translation Table

For displays on a black-and-white monitor, we need only one gray scale to assign a brightness intensity to a pixel according to its number of counts. The color monitor makes use of a look-up table to assign colors or different intensities of the same color to each pixel as a function of the pixel counts. Recall that a color on the monitor results from mixing together the three primary colors - red, green and blue. Any color in the visible light spectrum can be produced by combining these three primary colors in different proportions. The color translation table is therefore made up of three intensity scales, one for each of the three colors. For a given number of counts in the pixel, the color translation table assigns to it a unique combination of three integers, corresponding to the intensity of each of the electron beams in the color monitor.

Unlike the gray scale for a black-and-white monitor, which always increases from zero to the maximum, usually 255, the intensity scale for a color gun does not have to span the entire range of pixel counts. It could start from a certain count level which does not have to be zero, rise to a peak at some pixel count which does not have to be the maximum pixel count in the image, and fall to zero again beyond that. Figure 6-12 shows a hypothetical color scale which results from adding together the intensity scales for the red, green, and blue primary colors. This particular color combination scheme makes the low-count pixels appear blue on the monitor, the high-count pixels red, and a variety of other colors for pixels with counts in between. By changing the intensity of each electron gun, different proportions of the primary colors are mixed together to represent a given number of counts in a pixel. As a result, the image will appear in a completely new set of colors.

There is still much controversy in the literature on selecting the best color scheme to display radionuclide images on the video monitor. In spite of the many attempts to search for an optimal color scheme on an objective scientific basis, the preferred color is determined based on the esthetic appearance of the image in that color and on the color preferrence of the person reading the im-

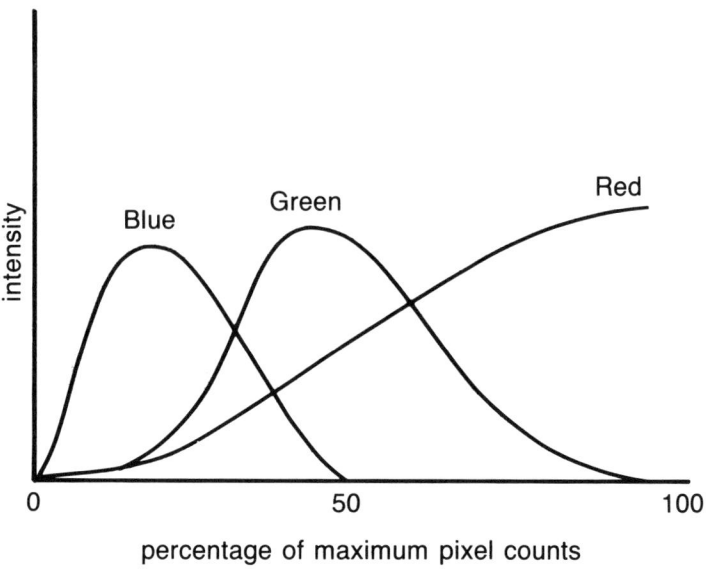

FIGURE 6-12 For a given pixel count, the color lookup table assigns one intensity to each of the three primary colors. The pixel color on the video monitor is a mixture of the three primary colors.

age. Whenever questions arise from interpreting the appearance of a radionuclide image in color, we tend to fall back on reading the same image in black-and-white. Perhaps one of the reasons for this practice is due to the physician's extensive experience with interpreting images on black and white film. Another reason could be attributed to the limited number of colors available in the average nuclear medicine computer display. In order to minimize the cost of the computer hardware, manufacturers typically limit their systems to display only 256 colors at any given time. Since our eyes are much more acute to a difference in colors than in shades of gray, we often hear complaints on the lack of continuity in a color image. Color display systems that can display over a million colors simultaneously on the monitor are now widely available and routinely used in the industry. Undoubtedly, such advanced color displays will become commercially available for routine display of nuclear medicine images in the near future. Also, as experience with interpreting color images accumulates, reliance on reading radionuclide images in black-and-white displays will become a thing of the past.

FRAME PROCESSING OPERATIONS

The frame processing operation is a pixel-by-pixel combination of two or more images to form one output image. The simplest example of frame operation is to add together several images acquired from a renogram to form one composite image in order to show clearly the shape and location of the kidneys. In this case, frame operation improves visualization of the kidneys by integrating a series of images to increase the count statistics.

Subtraction of an image pair is another example of frame processing, which forms the basis of digital subtraction angiography in radiology. An x-ray image is taken before the injection of a contrast agent into the blood vessel of the patient and another image is taken after injection. The preinjection image is subsequently subtracted from the postinjection image to produce a high contrast display of only those unobstructed vessels that permitted the contrast agent to pass through.

Another example is use of $^{201}Tl/^{99m}Tc$ for visualization of the parathyroid glands. Thallium-chloride is taken up by both the thyroid and the parathyroid glands, while pertechnetate is taken up only by the thyroid. If the patient is given both ^{201}Tl and ^{99m}Tc, one image could be taken with the window set at the 75-keV peak of ^{201}Tl and another image taken with the window over the 140-keV peak of ^{99m}Tc. Subsequently, subtraction of the ^{99m}Tc image from the ^{201}Tl image shows only the parathyroid glands in the resulting image. Usually, a few additional image manipulation steps are taken to equalize the number of counts in the two images before subtraction, but these details will not be discussed here.

GEOMETRIC OPERATIONS

Geometric operations are image processing functions that change the position or arrangement of the pixels in the image matrix. (For example, the two images to be subtracted are slightly shifted from one frame to another due to patient motion). Prior to subtraction, it is necessary to re-align the pixels in one image with respect to the other, both horizontally and vertically, until the reference marks on the patient coincide. Also, the ability of rotating an image about an arbitrary point to a specified angle is sometimes necessary to align the image pairs before subtraction. These types of geometric operations do not receive as much limelight as the smoothing and contrast enhancement operations because they do not require any exotic mathematical manipulations. Nevertheless, all are indispensible operations in every nuclear medicine system.

Other processing operations under the category of geometric operations are image magnification and minification. Magnification or minification of an image, after it has already been acquired, does not improve spatial resolution. During data acquisition, magnification may improve spatial resolution because the incoming counts are spaced out over a larger number of pixels according to their geometric locations instead of having them all crammed into a few big pixels. Unfortunately, after an image has been acquired, the exact coordinates of each count within a pixel are lost. Magnification of the image will not regain the original spatial information for each count; it only stretches out pixel counts over a wider area by interpolation. Therefore magnification or minification of an image that has already been acquired only makes it appear bigger or smaller, but does nothing to improve its spatial resolution.

CONCLUSION

Several fundamental concepts of image processing, specifically those pertinent to enhancement of the radionuclide images and the methods used to achieve them, have been introduced. Since radionuclide studies have become increasingly dependent on the computer for the extraction of qualitative and quantitative information, it is important for the user to master the concepts and goals of image processing and to become proficient with the techniques of digital manipulation of image data. The materials presented in this chapter will hopefully give the reader a basic understanding of digital image processing and pave the way for more in-depth perusal on selected topics of image processing in the literature.

SUGGESTED READINGS

1. Miller TR, Sampathkumaran KS. Digital filtering in nuclear medicine. *J Nucl Med* 1982;23:66-72.

2. Ram G. Optimization of ionizing radiation usage in medical imaging by means of image enhancement techniques. *Med Phys* 1982;9:733-737.

3. Todd-Pokpropek A. Image processing in nuclear medicine. *IEEE Trans Nucl Sci* 1980;NS27:1080-1094.

CHAPTER

7

QUANTITATIVE IMAGE ANALYSIS

INTRODUCTION

If the virtue of nuclear medicine amid competing imaging modalities is its ability to evaluate physiologic functions, then the justification for the existence of a nuclear medicine computer is its ability to perform quantitative evaluation of physiologic data obtained from the patient. The various image smoothing and contrast enhancement techniques are interesting and at times absolutely necessary, but the importance of these operations are only secondary to quantitative analysis of physiologic data.

One interesting characteristic common to the great majority of quantitative analyses, whether they are static or dynamic studies, is that they all strive toward calculating a numerical index as a gauge of an organ's physiologic function. In fact, many of these numerical indexes have become common terms—cardiac ejection fraction, V/Q ratio of the lungs, Q_p/Q_s ratio of cardiac shunts, effective renal plasma flow, etc.

Additionally, several computer operations are common to a large number of quantitative function studies. The quantification procedure involves drawing a region of interest (ROI) on the radionuclide image, calculating the number of counts within the ROI, and plotting a curve using the number of counts within the ROI as a function of time. Based on the activity versus time curve, one or more numerical indices of the organ's function are then derived.

CREATING ROIs

Drawing an ROI is one of the first steps in almost every image quantification operation. The ROI is usually the outline of an organ whose physiologic function is to be assessed by quantifying the amount of activity passing into or out of the region. Outlining the organ of interest is necessary because we only want to quantify the amount of activity within the organ under investigation and not within the other anatomic structures included in the field of view of the gamma camera.

Common ways of drawing an ROI are through the use of a joystick, a track ball, a light pen, or a mouse. Each one of these methods has its own nice features and frustrating moments, but with practice an ROI of any shape can be drawn equally well with any of the above devices. Drawing an ROI is initiated with the computer generating a dot or a cursor on the monitor. As the cursor is driven to different positions on the screen by the joystick, for instance, a line is traced out by the cursor to form the ROI.

Since the purpose of the ROI is to isolate the activity within the organ under investigation for quantification, the resulting ROI should be an accurate representation of the true edges of the organ. For studies such as the renogram, the operator can easily use visual judgement to move the cursor on the screen to create the desired ROI because the target-to-non-target count ratio is high and we are only interested in the relative change in the number of counts within the ROI from one image frame to another.

As a rule, however, organ boundaries are poorly defined in the vast majority of radionuclide images due to problems with camera-computer system resolution, organ motion, low organ uptake ratio, and overlapping activities in neighboring organs, etc. Under such circumstances, the visual judgement as to where to draw the organ outline can become exceedingly difficult. The subjective nature of visual judgement and drawing skill also make the resulting ROI highly variable between operators.

Subtracting a certain number of background counts from the image helps to increase image contrast and is frequently used to enhance organ visualization edges prior to manual drawing of the ROI by the operator. Alternatively, the operator can impose a count threshold on the gray scale to achieve nearly the same visual effect on the video display monitor as the actual subtraction of the background activity. However, these two operations must be used with caution. In many low-count and low-contrast images such as the gallium and delayed thallium studies, the background may be as high as 50%- 60% of the maximum pixel counts in the ROI. Excessive thresholding or background subtraction arbitrarily may underestimate organ size. Contrast enhancement by the convolution or Fourier techniques are seldom used to preprocess the image, not only because of the time factor but because of the possibility of producing distortions in the output images that may adversely affect the accuracy of the ROI. With some low-count images, smoothing the image with a nine-point filter after background subtraction is sometimes used to reduce statistical noise.

Due to the poor quality of some clinical images and the time and human subjectivity and variability involved with manually drawing ROIs, a number of computer algorithms have been devised with the aim of precisely identifying the organ edge objectively and consistently. These algorithms are commonly known as *automatic edge detection methods*.

Most automatic edge detection methods make use of the first or second derivative of the activity profiles to estimate the organ boundaries. While the actual computation procedure is rather involved, Figure 7-1 provides a conceptual understanding of the method. Figure 7-1A shows the activity profile across a slice of an organ. Just as we would expect intuitively, the activity profile changes little along the interior of the organ. But as we approach the edge of the organ, the curve drops off rapidly to the background level. Therefore, one criterion is to search for the edge of an organ in the pixel location where the activity profile shows the steepest decline. There is now a number, namely the slope of the activity profile, to assist us in finding the edge of the organ.

Instead of assessing the steepness of the activity profile at the various points by visual inspection, the first derivative curve (aslo known as a slope or gradient) as shown in Figure 7-1B is derived from the activity profile to show us quantitatively the rate at which the counts are changing. In our example, the numerical value of a point in the first derivative curve is the rate of change of the counts in the activity profile, when calculated in the direction from Point A towards Point E. The curve rises rapidly from zero to a maxi-

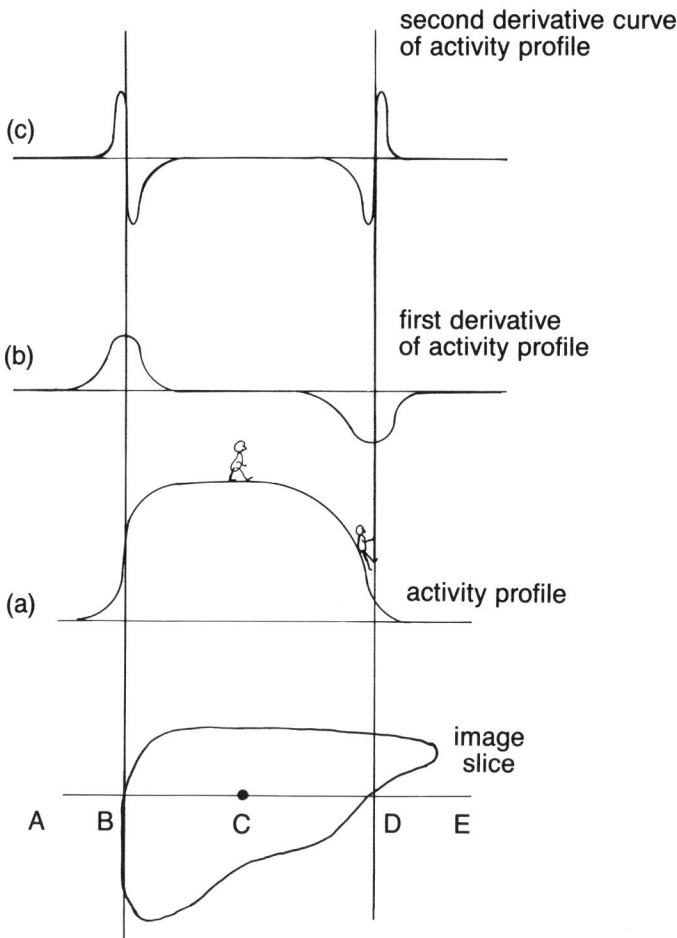

FIGURE 7-1 The second deriviative method for finding the intersecting points between the organ edges and the line AE.

mum at Point B, decreases to zero at Point C in the middle of the organ slice, and then changes rapidly to a minimum at Point D before returning to zero. This peculiar shape of the first derivative curve is due to the direction chosen to measure the slope of the activity profile. In moving along the activity profile from Point A towards Point B, the activity increases rapidly. The most rapid change occurs when crossing the boundary and entering the organ at Point B. This location corresponds to the location of the peak in the first derivative curve. Counts in the activity profile continue to increase after Point B, but at a slower pace. This is the reason why the first derivative curve drops after the peak at Point B. The mid-portion of the first derivative curve is close to zero because the activity distribution in the interior of the organ is relatively constant and does not change appreciably. As we approach Point D, the first derivative curve becomes increasingly negative because each point in the activity profile gives a fewer number of counts.

The minimum point in the first derivative curve corresponds to the pixel in the activity profile with the fastest rate of drop in counts. To elaborate further, the minimum point in the first derivative curve in Figure 7-1B has the fastest rate of decline of activity. The image pixel corresponding to the minimum, i.e., the most negative, point in the first derivative curve is where the counts drop off most rapidly. Other points located before and after the minimum are dropping off in counts too, but not as rapidly as the point with the maximum negative slope.

The gradient method for edge detection makes the fundamental assumption that the edge of an organ is where the pixel shows the most rapid change in counts. Physically, this assumption makes sense if we think of the edge of an organ as a thin membrane. This membrane separates the interior of the organ containing a high level of radioactivity on one side and the low-level background activity on the other side. The location of the membrane therefore corresponds to the transition point where the counts change rapidly from a very high to a very low value. This transition point is either the maximum or minimum point in the first derivative curve and is assumed to be the edge of the organ.

Since we are devising an algorithm to detect the edge automatically, without human intervention, we could instruct the computer to look for the maximum and minimum points in the first-derivative curve. The maximum and minimum points in the first-derivative curve would then correspond to the edges of the organ. However, most edge detection programs utilize the second-derivative curve instead of the first-derivative to aid in the identification of the organ edges. In an idealized example as shown in Figure 7-1, the second-derivative curve is almost symmetrical at the borders with two sharp peaks, thus making it easy for the computer to locate the edges. Also, the zero points on the second-derivative curve correspond to the maximum and minimum points on the first derivative curve. In most edge-detection programs, this zero point is automatically selected as the first approximation of the edge point.

However, due to the statistical noise, low contrast, and vague borders of radionuclide images, the true edge could be located anywhere from the zero point to the maximum point in the second-derivative curve. The minimum point on the second-derivative curve is not used because the corresponding pixel is located in the interior of the organ and using it as the edge would underestimate the size of the organ. In case the zero point does not correlate reasonably well with the true edge as assessed by visual judgment, the programs usually allow the user to specify a different second derivative value and to try again until a satisfactory edge point is found.

The same procedure can be repeated by constructing an activity profile for each row of pixels that pass through the organ of interest and determine the edge points according to the second derivative value. These points are then connected together as an ROI to represent the organ edge. Unfortunately, such a straightforward procedure for determining all the points needed to complete the ROI is time consuming. Most automatic edge detection programs begin with the computer asking the operator to position a rough ROI, such as a rectangle, over the organ whose edge is to be determined. The computer then draws eight equal-angle radii from the geometric center of the rectangle as shown in Figure 7-2. For each radius, the second derivative at each pixel location is calculated from the center and works out. As a first estimate, the point with a zero second-derivative value is chosen as an edge point. After all eight points (locations of zero second-derivative value) have been determined, another set of eight radii are drawn between the original ones, and the procedure is repeated to find the next eight edge points. Depending on the size of the organ, a sufficient number of points is usually generated to draw a continuous ROI after repeating the procedure two to three times. The algorithm described above is simplified to illustrate the central ideas behind the second-derivative edge detection method. The actual clinical programs used for automatic edge detection involve many more subtle details, such as background subtraction, thresholding, and smoothing on the image, in order to derive an ROI as close to the true edge of the organ as possible. How good are ROIs generated by automatic edge detection methods?

QUANTITATIVE IMAGE ANALYSIS 133

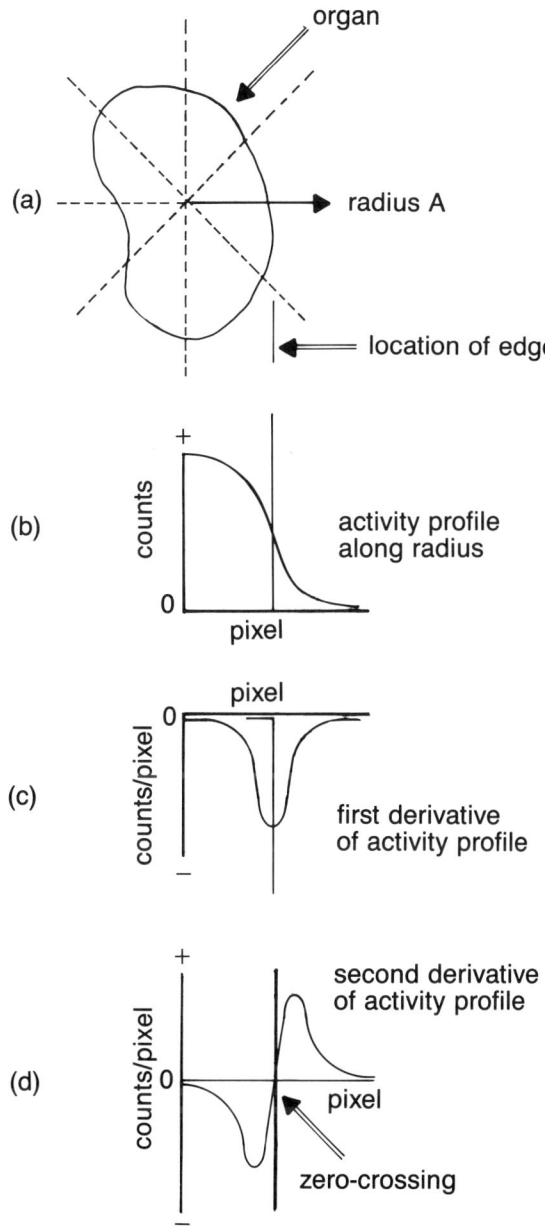

FIGURE 7-2 The 0-crossing of the second derivative of the activity profile is used as a point in the edge of the organ.

The automatic edge detection algorithms perform admirably well for organs with high uptake and good target-to-background ratios. For images with a low target-to-background ratio, such as those obtained from cardiac blood-pool studies with poor tagging, the computer-generated ROI can be erratic. For these types of images, some background subtraction is needed to increase the organ contrast. Nine-point image smoothing is also done to suppress the image noise prior to finding the edge with the automatic program. For some images in gated blood-pool studies, the separation of the left ventricle from the septum and the valve plane is so poor that we have to fall back on hand-drawing and use functional images such as the stroke volume image and the phase image as a guide.

One definite benefit in using automatic edge detection methods is the consistency of computer-generated ROIs. If the radionuclide has fairly good statistics and once the protocol for using the automatic edge detection program is determined, the same ROI is created each and every time no matter who the operator is. This consistency is valuable when we do sequential or follow-up studies. The aim there is to look for the direction of change in the physiologic state of the organ rather than the absolute value of some numerical index calculated for the organ. Of course, for noisy images, the ROI generated by the automatic edge detection method can vary widely from one trial to another, due to inconsistencies in the data.

CURVE GENERATION AND ANALYSIS

In many dynamic radionuclide studies, e.g., brain flow, renogram, and cardiac shunt studies, we are more interested in the flow characteristics of the tracer than visualization of the anatomical details of the involved organ. The starting point for analyzing the flow pattern quantitatively is the construction of an activity-versus-time curve, a plot of the number of counts within the ROI as a function of time. The resulting activity-versus-time curve is then used to derive one or more numerical indices to assess the physiologic function of the organ.

However, quantitative curve analyses can be difficult if there are big fluctuations in the curve data resulting from such problems as inconsistencies in the drawing of the ROI, poor count statistics, and other variabilities of real-world measurements. Unless the extreme statistical noise is removed from the data, the underlying information may become distorted.

Consider the data for the activity profile of a hypothetical radionuclide image as shown in Figure 7-3. A plot of the raw data as shown by Curve A shows the variation of the counts across a row of pixels in the image. If the curve data were to be analyzed quantitatively, more consistent results would be obtained if the noise appearing as local irregularities in the curve was removed.

One way to reduce the noise in the curve data is by performing a curve-smoothing operation. The simplest of all curve-smoothing operations is by *eye-balling* the original plot and drawing a smooth freehand curve through the data points. This eye-balling method offers a simple and convenient way to suppress local fluctuations in the curve data, but it has two distinct disadvantages. The eye-balling method is amenable to paper and pencil calculations, but much time and human effort are involved. In order to eye-ball a smooth curve, the computer or the human operator has to plot the original data on a sheet of graph paper, draw a smooth curve freehand by trial and error, read the new coordinates off the smooth

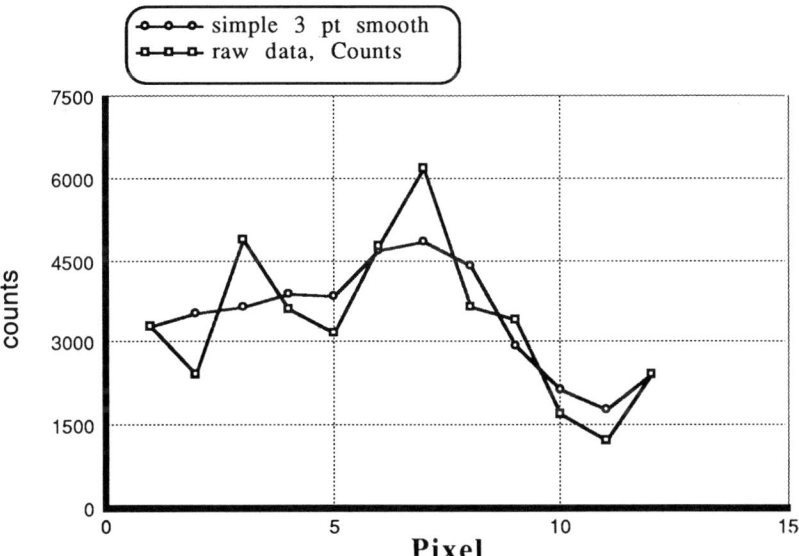

FIGURE 7-3 The effect of applying a simple three-point smoothing on a raw data curve.

curve, and then re-enter them into the computer. This laborious process is not feasible in any clinical environment. The second and even more serious deficiency is that the eye-balled value may not be statistically valid due to human bias. Fortunately, there are many other mathematical smoothing techniques that we can implement easily on the computer. The principles behind these curve smoothing techniques are similar to eye-balling, but the smoothing operation can be easily and objectively accomplished by the computer.

The Moving Average Method

The moving average method for curve smoothing is similar to the replace average method for spatial smoothing of radionuclide images. One example of a moving average algorithm is the three-point smooth, whereby the numerical value of a point of interest is replaced by the average of the data point itself and its two neighbors. That is,

$$Y_{new} = \frac{Y(n-1) + Y(n) + Y(n+1)}{3}$$

in fancy mathematical notation,

$$Y_{new} = \frac{1}{3} \sum_{i=n-1}^{n+1} Y_i$$

where Y(new) is the new smoothed value at point n, Y(n) is the original numerical value at that point, while $Y(n-1)$ and $Y(n+1)$ are the data points before and after Y(n), respectively. The new smoothed value is not used for the computation of the next average. Instead, the smoothed data are kept in a separate table; only the original data are used for calculating the moving average. The results of applying the three-point moving average to the curve data are given in Figure 7-3 and plotted as Curve B.

This example illustrates two common features of using the moving average method for curve smoothing. First, the moving average technique tends to smooth out extreme fluctuations in the data. Second, the first and the last data points are not generally averaged because each of these points has data on only one side.

QUANTITATIVE IMAGE ANALYSIS

The number of data points included in the moving average can be any odd number starting from three and on up (3, 5, 7, 9, ... etc.). For example, if a five-point moving average were used, the expression becomes

$$Y_{new} = \frac{Y(n-2) + Y(n-1) + Y(n) + Y(n+1) + Y(n+2)}{5}$$

Again, in elegant mathematical formalism, Ynew is expressed as

$$Y_{new} = \frac{1}{5} \sum_{i=n-2}^{n+2} Y_i$$

Note that only odd number of points are used in order to keep the smoothed points from being biased towards one direction of the curve. The smoothed data using a five-point average are plotted in Figure 7-4.

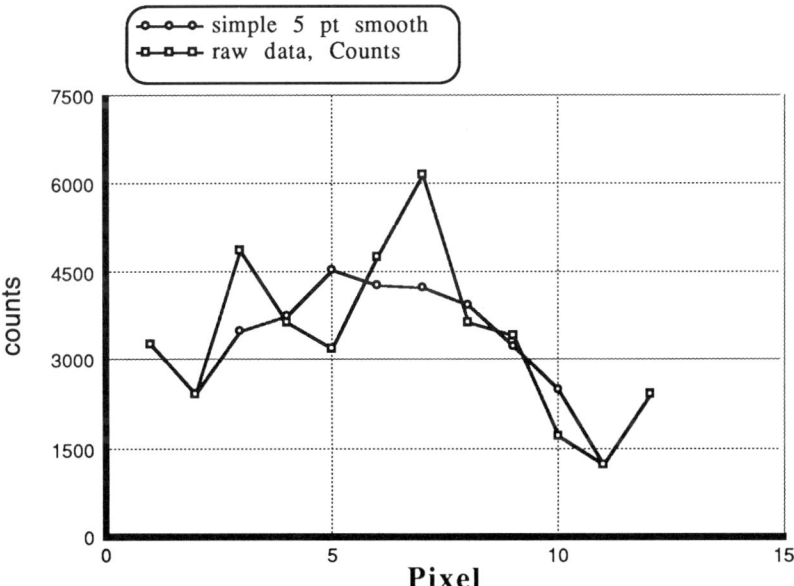

FIGURE 7-4 The effect of applying a simple five-point smoothing on a raw data curve.

The results derived from applying the three-point and five-point moving average are different. It is readily seen in Figure 7-4 that the five-point smoothed curve shows much greater suppression of the local fluctuations, while the three-point smoothed curve retains more of its local characteristics. In general, a greater amount of curve smoothing will result from averaging over a greater number of points in the curve. We should be aware that a smoother curve does not necessarily imply that it is more representative of the truth. And, just the contrary, over-smoothing a curve actually does more harm by damping out true local variations. In dynamic radionuclide studies, a three-point smooth is generally adequate to reduce the random fluctuations without excessively smoothing out true local variations.

The Weighted Moving-Average Method

The underlying assumption of the moving-average method implies that data from both sides of the point of interest, no matter how far away, have equal importance. We know intuitively, however, that the importance of a data point diminishes as its distance from the point of interest increases. Therefore, the problems caused by averaging over a large number of curve points can be partially alleviated by applying a weight to each point. The weighted average method is stated mathematically as follows:

$$Y_{new} = \frac{1}{\sum w_i} \sum w_i Y_i$$

where $i = 1, 2, 3,..$ etc, and w_i is the weight or weighting coefficient applied to a given point. The subscript i indicates the number of places that the given point is displaced from the point of interest. Thus, for a five-point smooth the subscript i takes on values of (-2, -1, 0, 1, 2), while a three-point smooth has values of (-1, 0, 1).

The simple moving average is actually a special case of the weighted-moving average where the weight $w_i = 1$ for all i. Curve data in nuclear medicine studies are typically smoothed using the weighted three-point average method and the weighting coefficients $w_{-1} = 1/4$, $w_0 = 1/2$, and $w_1 = 1/4$. These weighting coefficients imply that the data on either side are only half as important as the

QUANTITATIVE IMAGE ANALYSIS 139

data at the point of interest itself. Figure 7-5 compares a curve smoothed by using a three-point weighted average with the above coefficients, a curve smoothed by a simple average with equal weights, and the original curve. It is readily seen that the weighted-average curve retains more of the characteristics of the original curve than the curve smoothed with the simple moving average.

Data Smoothing by Curve Fitting

The weighted and nonweighted moving-average methods treat local fluctuations in the curve data as random noise. The averaging operations are attempts to smooth out statistical noise by making each point take a more gradual transition from its neighbors. These methods make no assumptions as to what particular curve pattern or mathematical function the data should follow. A more sophisticated method for data smoothing, regression analysis, assumes that the curve data conform to a certain mathematical function. The regression or least-squares curve fitting procedure is the analytic

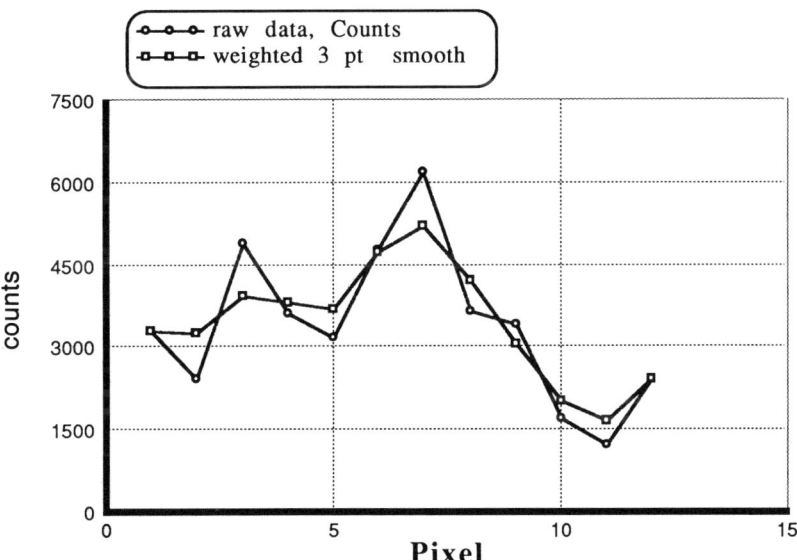

FIGURE 7-5 The effect of applying a weighted three-point smoothing on a raw data curve.

method to derive the parameters of the desired function that the resulting equation will describe the curve data with the least amount of error.

The linear least-squares curve fitting procedure is perhaps the most familiar example. Here, we assume that data follow a straight line function in the form of

$$Y(x) = A + Bx,$$

where $Y(x)$ and x are the dependent and independent variables, respectively. A is called the Y-intercept and is a constant equal to the value of $Y(x)$ when $x = 0$, and B is another constant equal to the slope of the straight line. A straight line is completely determined once the slope B and the Y-intercept A are found.

The least-squares curve fitting criterion is to look for the best values for the slope B and the intercept A that the sum of the square of the difference between the calculated $Y(x)$ and the original data $Y(n)$ is at a minimum. Since the exact mathematical operations to calculate the desired parameters A and B are described in all introductory statistics text, they will not be repeated here.

When we eye-ball a smooth curve through the raw data, we are actually performing a least-squares curve fitting using our visual judgement. Unfortunately, the eye-balling method lacks objectivity and we may not be certain that the eye-balled curve is the one that gives the minimum error between the raw data and the calculated values.

Linear least-squares curve fitting is applicable to a wide variety of curve data. Data that do not follow a straight line in the original plot may become linear after appropriate transformation. For example, radioactivity decreases exponentially with time. When the activity in a sample is plotted as a function of time (Fig. 7-6), a familiar exponential curve is obtained. However, the exponential curve becomes a straight line in a semi-log plot in Figure 7-7 when the logarithm of the activity is plotted as a function time. The reason is obvious because the equation for radioactive decay:

$$A = A_o e^{-\lambda \tau}$$

after a logarithmic transformation becomes

$$\log A = \log (A_o) - \lambda t$$

If we let $Y = \log A$, $A = \log (A_o)$, and $Bx = \lambda t$, then $Y = A + Bx$, which is the form of a straight line in a semi-log plot. Thus, most of the exponential curve fitting procedures found in nuclear medicine software package are merely an extension of the linear least-squares curve fitting procedure by first doing a logarithmic transform of the dependent variable, e.g., the number of counts within a ROI.

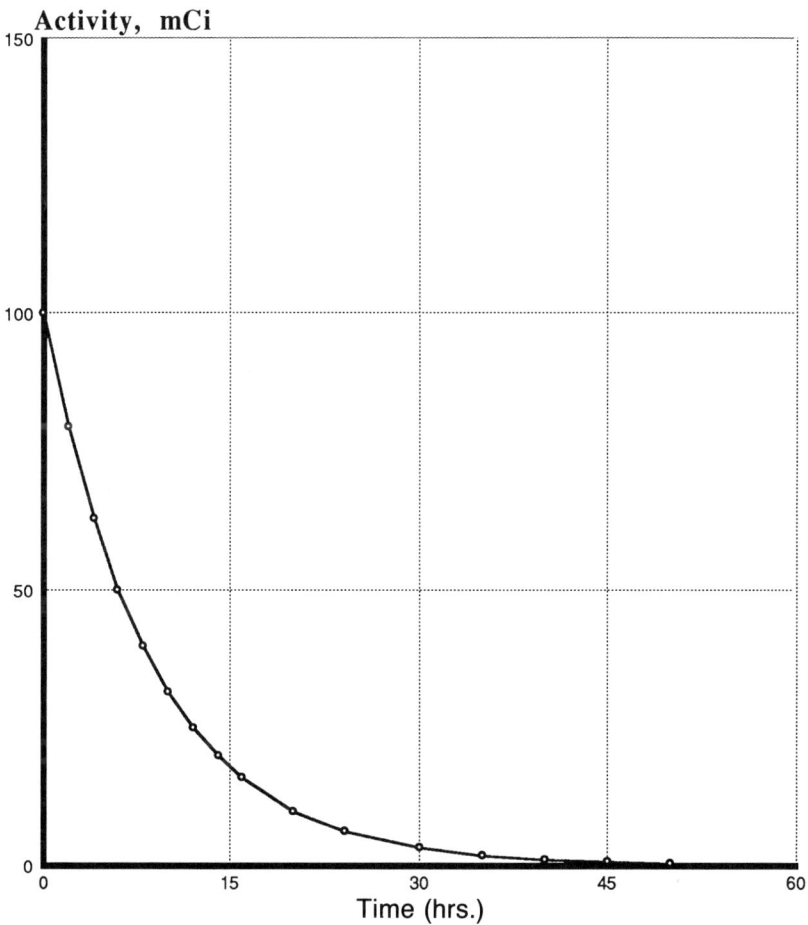

FIGURE 7-6 The decay curve of ^{99m}Tc in a linear plot.

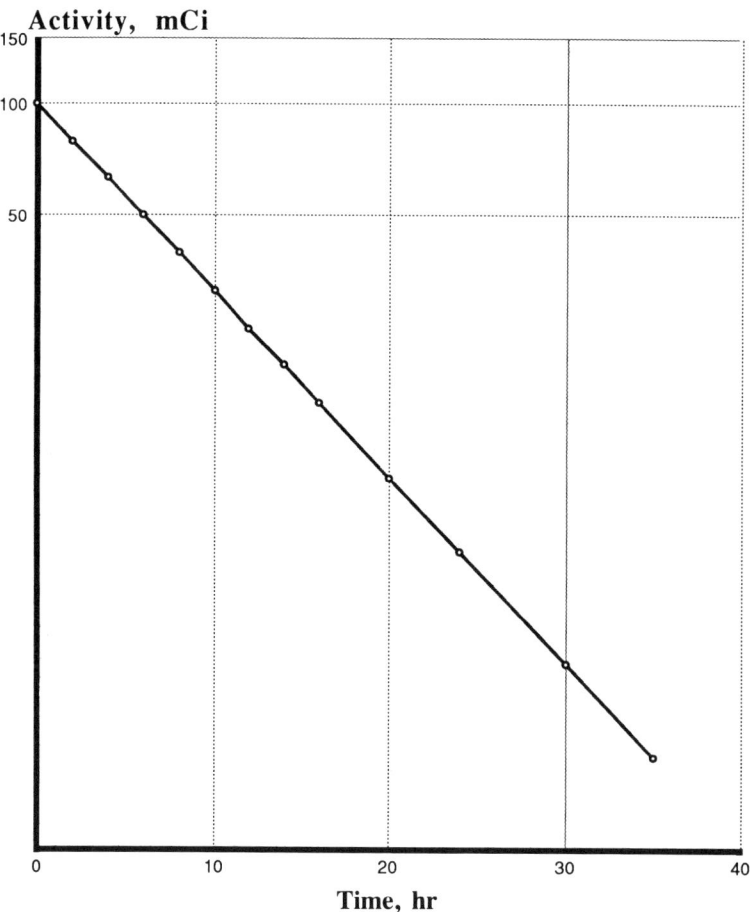

FIGURE 7-7 The decay curve of ^{99m}Tc in a semi-log plot.

Likewise, the radiation intensity when measured at various distances from a point source drops off as an inverse square function of the distance. According to Figure 7-8, a plot of the measured activity as a function of distance yields a hyperbolic curve. However, when the logarithm of the measured intensity is plotted as a function of the logarithm of the distance as in Figure 7-9, a straight line is obtained. The equation for the inverse squared relationship between the measured radiation intensity and distance is:

$$I\ d^2 = K,$$

QUANTITATIVE IMAGE ANALYSIS 143

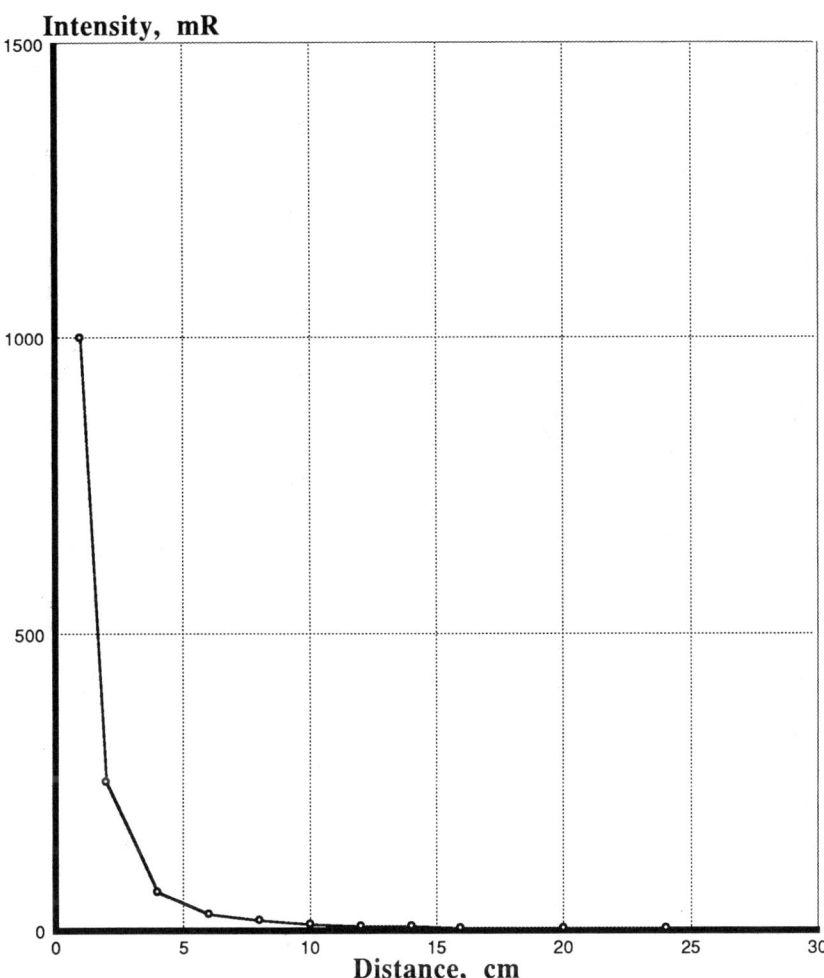

FIGURE 7-8 The reduction of radiation intensity as a function of distance from a point source in a linear plot.

where I is the measured activity, K is an arbitrary constant, and d is the distance from the source. Taking the logarithm of the two sides of the equation, we get:

$$\log I + 2 \log d = \log K$$

or

$$\log I = \log K - 2 \log d.$$

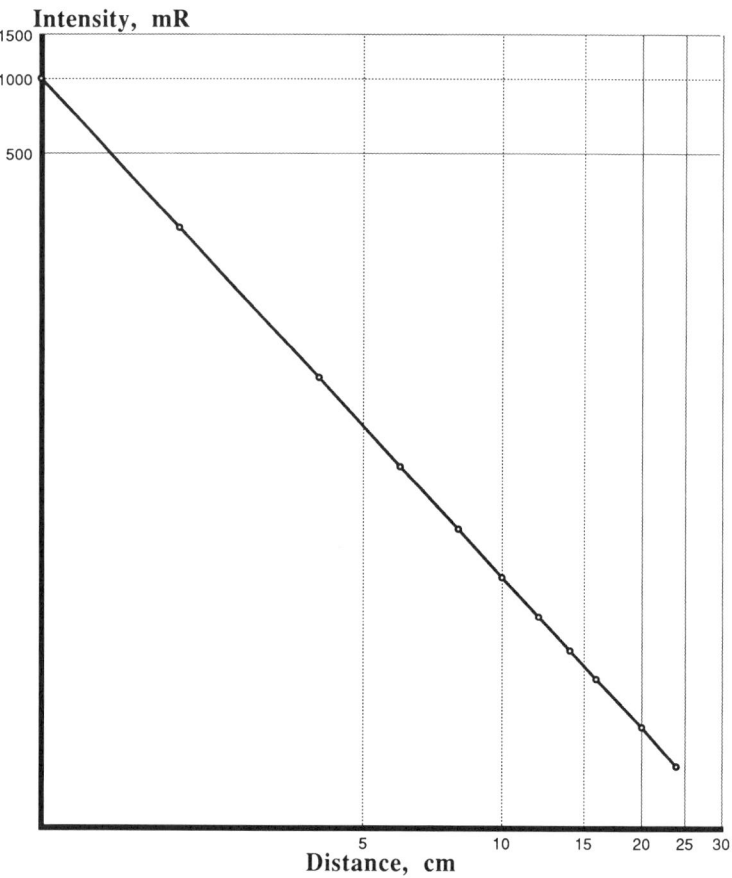

FIGURE 7-9 The reduction of radiation intensity as a function of distance from a point source in a linear plot.

Again, if we let Y = log I, A = log K, B = -2, and x = log d, we obtain the equation Y = A + Bx is obtained, which is the expression for a straight line in a log-log plot.

However, for curves that do not change monotonically in one direction, a linear least-squares fitting is inappropriate. For example, the volume curve obtained from a gated ventricular blood-pool study is fitted with a cosine curve as shown in Figure 7-10, or the 3rd order polymonial if you want to examine the systolic and diastolic indices; and the lung-activity curve for cardiac shunt studies are analyzed by fitting the original data to two gamma functions to characterize the pulmonary and systemic flows as shown in Figure 7-11. In these two examples of non-linear least-squares curve fitting, we attempt to find a mathematical equation of the desired form that will minimize the sum of the squares of the differences between the raw data and the calculated value. These details will be discussed fully in Chapter 8.

Miscellaneous Curve Manipulation Techniques

There are many other curve arithmetic operations such as the integration of the area under a curve between two points and the addition, subtraction, multiplication, and division of a curve by a constant or by another curve. These arithmetic operations are simple and their action on the curve data is obvious so they will not be described here, but they nevertheless are indispensible in nuclear medicine software.

CONCLUSION

Writing a computer program for curve smoothing, edge detection, or compartmental analysis of physiologic functions is simple. Choosing the mathematical models, curve-fitting parameters, and criter-

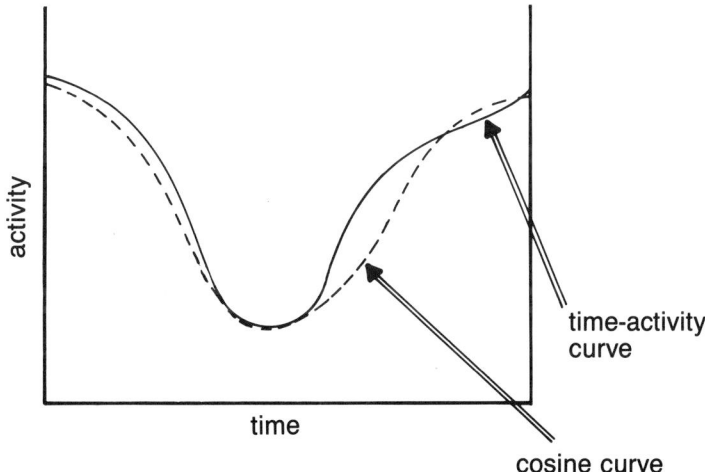

FIGURE 7-10 The least-squares fitting of the cardiac volume curve to a cosine function.

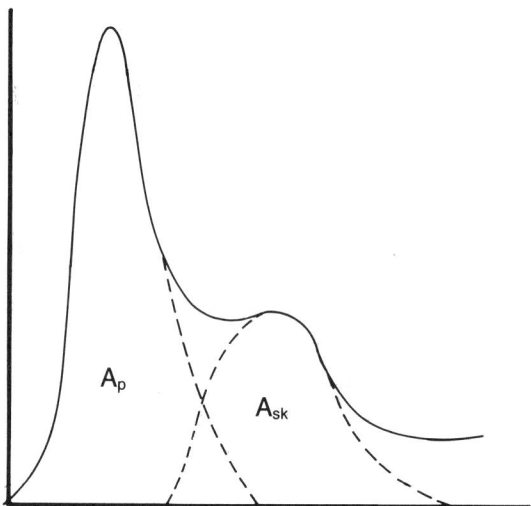

FIGURE 7-11 The time-activity curve of the lungs is fitted with two gamma functions.

ia for judging the goodness of fit is difficult. The computer is convenient and objective, but its computations are vulnerable to noise in the data and deviation of the patient data from assumptions used in the mathematical model. Therefore, do not trust everything the computer tells you. Eyeballing and common sense are still the best tools for keeping the computer honest!

SUGGESTED READINGS

1. Rabinowitz A, Wexler JP, Blaufox MD. Quantification of the radionuclide images. Theorectical concepts and the role of the computer. In: Freeman LM, ed. *Clinical radionuclide imaging.* New York: Grune and Stratton; 1984:261-313.
2. Rosner B. *Fundamentals of biostatistics,* second edition. Boston: Duxbury Press; 1986.
3. Savitzky A, Golay MJE. Smoothing and differentiation of data—simplified least-squares procedure. *Anal Chem 1964*; 36:1627-1639.

CHAPTER

8

NUCLEAR CARDIOLOGY

INTRODUCTION

Since their modest beginning in the early 1970s, cardiac studies comprise nearly one-third of the total procedures done in nuclear medicine today. In fact, the maturation of the dynamic blood-pool technique in the mid-1970s as an accurate, convenient and noninvasive procedure for evaluating cardiac function legitimatizes the computer as an integral piece of equipment for every nuclear medicine department.

Radionuclide cardiac studies are divided into three categories: (1) multiple-gated equilibrium, (2) first-pass blood-pool, and (3) static myocardial perfusion studies. The discussion will focus upon the various analytical and and computer methods that have been developed for the evaluation of multiple-gated blood-pool studies because many of the same techniques are directly applicable to the analysis of the first-pass studies. For completeness, methods for quantifying the myocardial perfusion studies only will be discussed briefly at the end of the chapter.

Usually any discussion of cardiac blood-pool studies begins with data acquisition methods. Traditionally, the list-mode acquisition method is identified with first-pass studies, while the multiple-gated frame mode acqusition method is associated with equilibrium blood-pool studies. Due to recent advances in the computer technology, such a generalization is no longer valid.

METHODS OF DATA ACQUISITION

List-Mode Acquisition

List mode acquisition is also known as serial mode acquisition. Recall that each count recorded by the gamma camera carries two numbers corresponding to the x and y coordinates of the scintillation event in the plane of the NaI crystal. In the case of frame-mode acquisition, the incoming counts are sorted into the respective pixels according to their x and y coordinates during the time of acquisition. Of course, a finite length of time is required by the computer to determine to which pixel in the image matrix an incoming count belongs. Once the pixel location is determined, another time interval is required to increment the total number of counts in that pixel by one. During the time the computer is busy sorting and incrementing counts into their respective pixels, the computer is not responsive to any additional counts from the gamma camera. For dynamic studies with a high transient counting rate, a number of counts could be lost during this computer deadtime.

List-mode acquisition shortens this computer deadtime by not performing any data sorting and arithmetics at the same time that the counts are being collected. Figure 8-1 shows that the x and y coordinates for each count are sequentially recorded in the buffer memory or on the disk as they arrive from the gamma camera. At regular time intervals, typically at 1 or 10 msec apart, a timing-mark is also registered to indicate the arrival time of the counts. This pattern of data recording means that the timing-marks are not necessarily spaced equally on the disk. The timing-marks can be separated far apart by a large number of counts when the count rate is high and placed closely together if only a few counts are recorded in an identical time interval. Keep in mind, however, that the elapsed time between any two consecutive timing-marks is always the same regardless of the number of counts recorded in between.

The maximum speed at which counts can be acquired in list mode depends on the rate of the analog-to-digital converter and the rate that the data can be written into the buffer memory or onto the disk. With modern high-speed memory and disk drives, counting rates in excess of 200,000 cps can be accomodated. However, the rate of data input to the computer is limited by the gamma

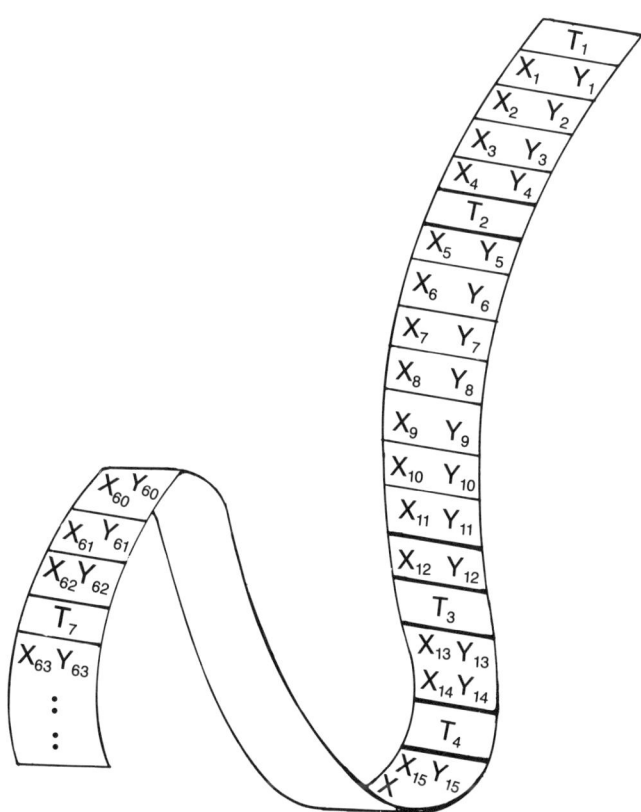

FIGURE 8-1 In list-mode acquisition, the x and y coordinates of each count is recorded sequentially in the computer. Typically, at every 10 msec, a timing mark is recorded to indicate arrival time of the counts.

camera, which at the current state-of-the-art can handle at the most 100,000 cps without a severe loss of image resolution.

Since the spatial resolution of a conventional 40-cm diameter gamma camera is limited to a 256 x 256 matrix, one byte (2^8 = 256) is sufficient for holding the largest numerical value of a coordinate. Thus, two bytes are needed to record one count. List mode acquisition is therefore incredibly hungry for storage space. You may recall that if we acquired a study using frame mode acquisition, one byte would be able to hold 255 counts. If the same acquisition was done in list mode, 255 counts would need 510 bytes of storage space!

To acquire a study of 50,000-70,000 counts, such as in a typical first-pass cardiac study, at least 100 KB to 140 KB of space would be needed.

Another shortcoming of list-mode acquisition is that several minutes of postacquisition time is required to sort the list of accumulated counts according to their x and y coordinates and place them into their respective pixels to form an image. In the case of frame-mode acquisition, the image is ready for viewing immediately upon termination of acquisition.

List-mode acquistion does offer several important advantages:

1. It has the ability to acquire data at a high transient counting rate with a minimum amount of data loss.
2. It offers a high temporal resolution as short as one millisecond to enable quantitative evaluation of rapid flows.
3. It allows the flexibility in selecting the counts to coordinate with the desired physiologic parameters for image reformatting. In fact, this third advantage is the main reason why list mode acquisition is still used in nuclear cardiology.

In spite of the advantages, however, the use of list mode alone for data acquisition is nearly extinct. Newer computers are able to perform frame-mode acquisition at 100 frames per second using a 64 x 64 matrix with a count rate of 200,000 cps, which is much faster than the highest count rate any single-crystal gamma camera is able to achieve. The current practice of nuclear cardiology acquires counts from the gamma camera by using the rapid dynamic frame-mode acquisition method for first-pass studies and a combination of the list-mode and multiple-gated frame modes for equilibrium blood-pool studies.

Multiple-Gated Acquisition

Multiple-gated acquisition is a special type of dynamic frame-mode acquisition that uses the electrocardiograph (ECG) signals from the patient to regulate the framing rate. Although multiple-gated acquisition is almost synonymous with dynamic blood-pool studies, it has been used with a small degree of success by gating the respiration cycles to reduce the lung motion artifacts during perfusion lung imaging.

A movie-making technique explains why such a complicated gating procedure is needed to acquire data for viewing heart motion. Suppose we want to take a snap shot of a high-speed car chase. We would need to set our camera to a fast shutter speed. Otherwise, the image of the moving cars will be blurred. To support such a high-shutter speed, a bright source of light is also necessary in order to get sufficient exposures on the film.

In data acquisition for a dynamic heart study, most computers have no trouble with acquiring counts in excess of 60 frames per second, probably the maximum framing rate necessary for capturing heart motion. Unfortunately, we would not be able to collect a sufficient number of counts from the cardiac blood pool to form an image at such a high framing rate. This problem is analogous to taking a snap shot at night of a fast-moving car, where there would be insufficient light to expose the film to the proper density. Unlike the case of the bad guy fleeing from the cops, the heart muscles return to the same location several tens of times per minute. Also, the heart informs us with a signal on the ECG machine at the onset of each contraction.

The multiple-gated acquisition method takes advantage of the cyclical motion of the heart and synchronizes the rate and direction of data acquisition with the ECG signals. This method is easy to understand with the aid of Figure 8-2. There, we arbitrarily break the cardiac cycle into 24 segments. Next, the computer is instructed to set aside enough space in the memory for 24 frames of image, each frame consisting of an matrix of 64 x 64 words. Some clinicians use a 128 x 128 matrix in order to obtain a higher spatial resolution. However, we can obtain the resolution of a 128 x 128 matrix by zooming the image two times bigger at the time of acquisition. The advantages of zooming are that the amount of computer memory and disk space required for storing the data is reduced and extraneous anatomic structures from the images are excluded.

Prior to acquiring data into the image matrices, the computer takes a sample of the R-waves from the ECG and calculates the average time interval between two consecutive R-waves. This average R-R time interval is assumed to be the time for each complete heart cycle. If we instruct the computer to set aside room in the memory

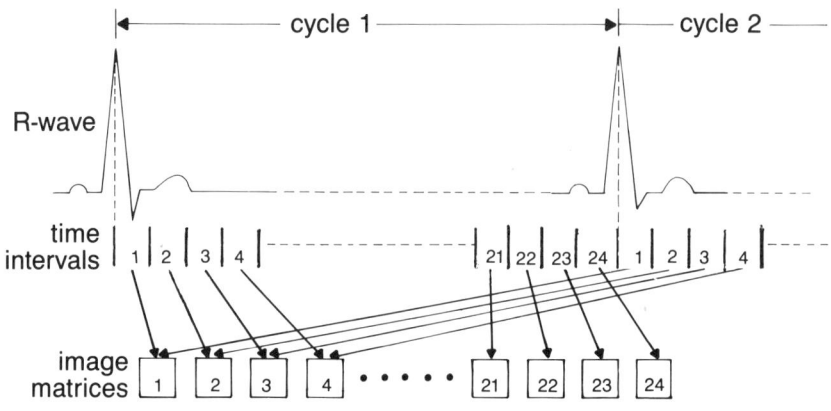

FIGURE 8-2 The R-wave from the ECG serves as the marker to sort data from the same phase of different heart cycles into one image frame.

for 24 frames of images, then the R-R time interval is correspondingly divided into 24 segments. For example, if the patient's heart rate is 72 bpm, then each heart beat or R-R time interval is 0.833 seconds long (60 seconds/72 beats). Upon dividing this 0.833 seconds R-R time interval into 24 segments, each segment is 35 msec long.

When data acquisition begins, the R-wave from the ECG triggers the computer to direct all incoming counts to be stored in Frame 1 for the next 35 msec. At the end of 35 msec, the computer then redirects the counts to be stored in Frame 2 for 35 msec, and so on. This same data acquisition pattern continues for each 35-msec segment until the arrival of the next R-wave, at which time the R-wave switches the computer back to Frame 1, and the whole cycle is repeated again. After 10 minutes of data acquisition, data from 720 heart beats will have been accumulated into 24 frames in the computer memory. Although the number of counts collected from each individual heart cycle is small, by accumulating counts from the same phase of the cardiac cycle into the same frame in the computer, 200,000 counts can be acquired into each frame with a 20-mCi dose. This set of 24 images shows the heart during the different phases of one complete cardiac cycle, each with sufficient number of counts accumulated from many hundred cardiac cycles to become statistically significant.

NUCLEAR CARDIOLOGY

Temporal Resolution

Before the initiation of the multiple-gated frame-mode acquisition, the user must decide into how many image frames will the data acquired from a cardiac cycle be divided. Here there is a compromise between two conflicting requirements: The desire for a high temporal resolution and low statistical noise. For a practical acquisition time, high temporal resolution can be obtained only at the expense of increased statistical noise.

For qualitative assessment of wall motion, a framing rate as low as 16 frames per cycle is probably sufficient. With too low a framing rate, the poor temporal resolution will produce disturbing flickers during cine display (like the old time jumpy movies). It may also underestimate the ejection fraction (EF) because the assumed end-systole frame may not correspond to the precise moment of maximum heart contractions. The trade-off here is that a high framing rate results in too few number of counts per image. As a result, statistical noise could produce a large fluctuation of the EF and fuzzy heart images during cinematic display of the image series. On the other hand, a low framing rate results in a loss of temporal resolution and produces flickering during cinematic display and underestimation of the EF due inaccurate identification of the end-systole (ES) phase of the cardiac cycle.

For the purpose of calculating EF and viewing wall motion, between 20-30 frames per cycle will yield sufficient temporal resolution and adequate count statistics for each frame. For quantitative analysis of the heart dynamics such as the peak ejection and filling rates, higher framing rates such as 40-70 frames per cycle are desirable for accurate determination of the slopes in the activity-versus-time curve.

Artifacts From Arrythmia

There is one major problem with the multiple-gated acquisition method for cardiac studies. The method assumes that the heart rate remains constant throughout the duration of the acquisition—10 minutes for most studies. For patients with irregular heart rates, an erratic heart beat may occur intermittently with the R-R time interval, either shorter or longer than previously calculated by the computer. The consequence of having too short a heart beat is illustrated in Figure 8-3. If the R-R interval is shorter than the one assumed by the computer, say 700 msec instead of 833 msec for the present example, the next R-wave arrives when the computer is still acquiring data into Frame 20 (20 frames x 35 msec/frame = 700 msec). The unexpected early arrival of the next R-wave resets the computer to put counts starting from Frame 1 again. As a result, Frames 21-24 miss all the counts from the last part of the cardiac cycle.

The consequence of an R-R interval longer than the one previously calculated by the computer is shown in Figure 8-4. Let us assume that the next R-R interval is 1.0 second instead of 0.833 second. The computer acquires data into each of the 24 frames at the rate of 35 msec per frame. If the computer finishes putting counts into Frame 24 and the next R-wave still has not arrived, the computer simply stops acquiring until it is reset by the arrival of the next R-wave. The consequence to the data is nearly the same as in the case of a short R-R time interval; the last several frames of the study show a drop in counts because the data were not recorded corresponding to the maximum filling phase of the ventricular cycle. Figure 8-5 compares the results of including R-R time intervals either longer or shorter than the reference value calculated by the computer at the beginning of the study. In some cases, the last several frames in the image series suffer loss of counts.

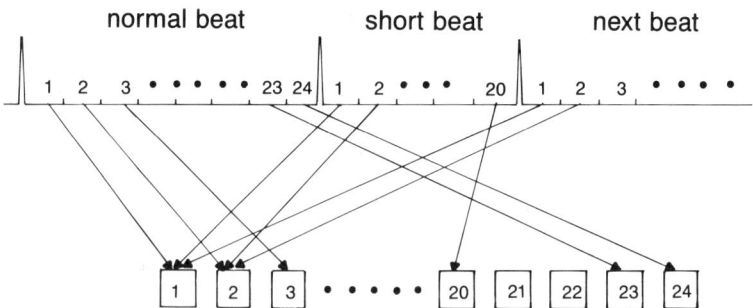

FIGURE 8-3 If an abnormal heart beat occurs while counts are accumulating in Frame 20, the unexpected R-wave resets the computer to direct incoming counts to Frame 1. No counts will be recorded in Frames 21-24 during this short cardiac cycle.

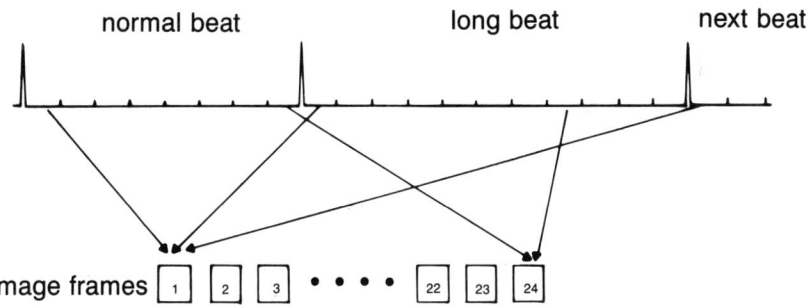

FIGURE 8-4 If an R-R interval lasts longer than the reference value, the last several image frames will be acquired before maximum filling. Hence, the ending frames will have fewer counts than the initial frames.

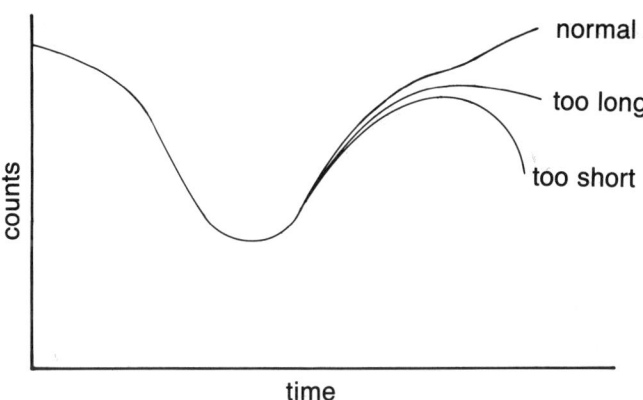

FIGURE 8-5 Comparison of the volume curves for multi-gated studies acquired with heartbeats longer or shorter than normal.

Buffered Gated-Beat Acquisition

Some computers attempt to solve arrhythymia problems by combining the frame and list modes into one acquisition sequence as illustrated in Figure 8-6. This method of gated acquisition reserves three areas in the buffer memory for data storage. One chunk of memory, Buffer 1, is reserved to hold a series of image frames, and the other two areas are reserved to store data in list mode. Before data ac-

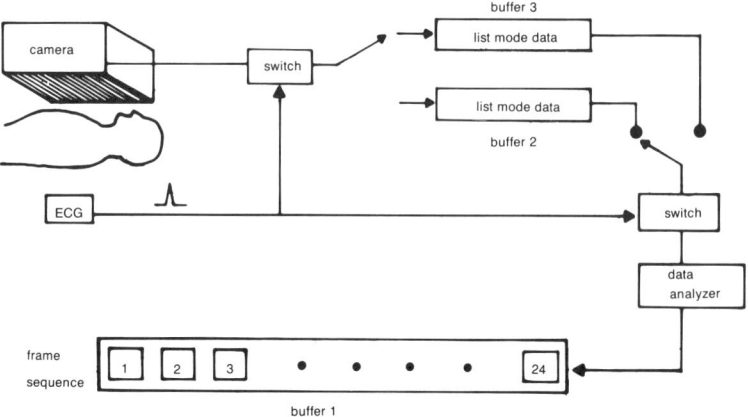

FIGURE 8-6 Buffered gating method records counts from each heartbeat in list mode. If the R-R interval is within the selected range, the counts will be reformatted and added onto the composite images in the frame buffer.

quisition, the computer displays a histogram of the R-R intervals and asks the operator to specify the acceptable range of R-R time intervals. Upon initiation of data acquisition and the detection of an R-wave, the incoming counts are stored in list mode in one of the temporary buffers, e.g., Buffer 2. When the second R-wave arrives, the incoming counts are switched to the other storage buffer, Buffer 3 in this example. While acquisition in Buffer 3 is conducted under the control of the acquisition processor, the central processing unit (CPU) measures the R-R time interval recorded in Buffer 2. If the beat length is within the specified range, the data are then added to the respective pixels in Buffer 1. The counts are ignored if the R-R interval of the previous heart beat is outside the acceptable range.

Thus, the area reserved in Buffer 1 is for accumulating data from all heart beats within the specified range of heart rates, while the other two areas in the list mode buffer are used alternately for temporary storage of only one heart beat's worth of data. Since the counting rate from an equilibrium blood-pool study is between 30,000-50,000 cps and the duration of one heart beat is approximately 1 second, the acquisition buffer should have at least 100,000 bytes (100 KB) of storage for holding data in each of the two list-

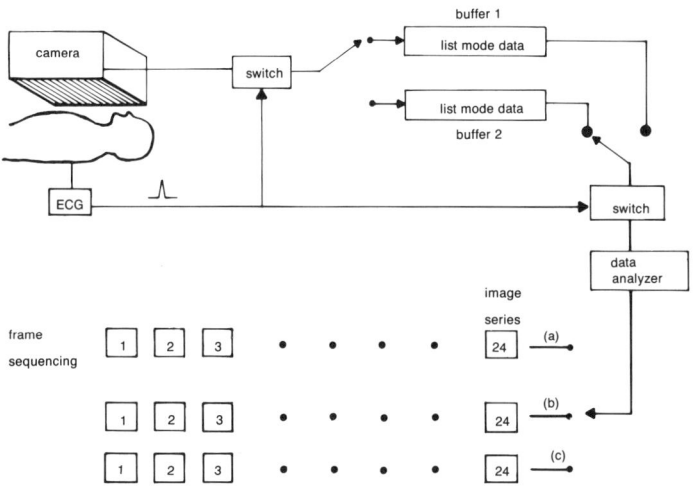

FIGURE 8-7 Multi-window buffered gated acquisition sorts counts from two or more ranges of R-R intervals to form corresponding series of images.

mode zones. Also, the CPU must be able to finish processing data from one heart beat before the completion of the second heart beat in order to avoid any data losses. Given the low cost of computer memory and the speed of the CPU, most computers will have no problem in satisfying these requirements.

As an extension of the single-beat length selection method, some computer software allows two or more windows of acceptable R-R time intervals as shown in Figure 8-7. Before acquisition starts, the computer measures the beat length for several minutes and then displays on screen a histogram of the beat lengths detected in that time interval. If the user decides, for example, to select three windows of acceptable R-R intervals, the computer will then set aside space in the buffer memory to hold three series of gated images. Upon initiation of data acquisition, counts will be alternately acquired into the temporary list-mode zones and then sorted into the corresponding image series, depending on the length of the R-R interval. The requirements for two or more concurrent multiple-gated studies are that the computer must have sufficient storage capacity to hold both the temporary and cumulative data and be able to sort the data fast enough to minimize data loss while performing the data sorting.

Again, state-of-the-art computers can easily meet these two requirements.

Artifacts From Delayed Gating

Count loss in the last several frames of a multiple gated image series is explained by R-R intervals that are either longer or shorter than the initially calculated value. If we have significant count losses in the first several frames of the image series, the problem is most likely caused by improper gating of the ECG signals. Ideally the first and the last few frames of the image series should have the highest and nearly the same number of counts because they represent the maximum filling of blood in the ventricles before contraction. The algorithm assumes that the R-wave is a signal for the onset of systole and that the ventricle is at its maximum filling. Most ECG-gating devices trigger the computer at the down slope of the R-wave to acquire counts starting at the first frame of the image series. If the ECG gate is delayed in sending out the trigger or if the computer is delayed in reacting to the trigger, the ventricular systole would start before the computer is able to begin acquisition. As a result, the first several frames have fewer counts than the last several frames because the images were acquired after the blood had started to empty from the ventricles. The problem is more acute with fast heart rates when the R-R time intervals are short and if the delay is a significant fraction of the R-R time interval. The result of delayed gating trigger is illustrated in Figure 8-8.

ANALYSIS OF MULTIPLE-GATED BLOOD-POOL IMAGES

Multiple-gated blood-pool studies are used a lot more frequently to assess ventricular function than first-pass studies. Of the many justifications given by the clinicians for their preference, those most frequently mentioned are:

1. The outcome of the study is not affected by the technique of injection and does not require precise coordination with the start of the computer acquisition.

2. Higher count statistics.
3. The ability to visualize the left ventricle from a number of different projections.
4. Only a single radionuclide injection is needed for sequential studies, such as multiple acquisitions at different levels of stress exercise.

Qualitative Data Analysis

One of the most effective ways to assess the cardiac contractility is by cyclically showing the series of multiple-gated images on the monitor in rapid succession to create a movie-like impression of a beating heart. Although this visual assessment of cardiac function is subjective, the magnitude and location of suspected wall motion abnormalities have been shown to correlate well with cine radiography. In fact, simultaneous movie display of the multiple gated images acquired from different projections is especially useful to pinpoint regions of abnormal wall contraction.

Due to the relatively poor count statistics of only 200,000 counts per image, several image manipulation processes are invariably done to improve the image quality prior to the cinematic display. Spatial, temporal smoothing, and count normalization are the three most

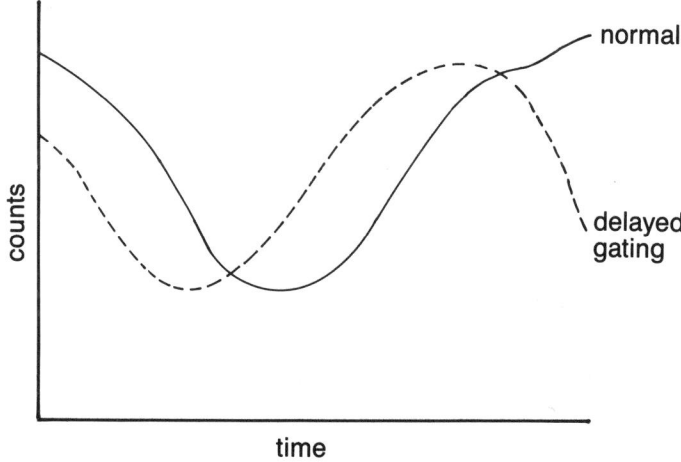

FIGURE 8-8 A volume curve with reduced counts at the beginning is most likely caused by delays in the computer or the ECG device.

frequently performed processes for image enhancement. For multiple-gated images, it is common for each frame in the series to be spatially smoothed by the nine-point weighted smoothing kernel below:

$$1/16 \begin{bmatrix} 1 & 2 & 1 \\ 2 & 4 & 2 \\ 1 & 2 & 2 \end{bmatrix}$$

The purpose of image smoothing is, of course, to reduce the high frequency noise. For low-contrast images, such as those acquired with poorly labeled blood pool and a heavy background activity, a number of background counts is subtracted from the image to increase the contrast. However, such an operation also reduces the total number of counts, resulting in a noisier image. Under such circumstances, images are smoothed more than once using the nine-point smoothing kernel to make the images appear more esthetically pleasing.

Temporal Smoothing

In clinical practice, we take 12-32 frames in one complete cycle of the cardiac blood pool. Temporal smoothing is usually applied to the image series to produce a gradual variation of counts from one frame to the next. Temporal smoothing reduces the amount of flickering by softening any abrupt changes in the pixel counts between frames. The number of counts in any given pixel of a frame, when temporally smoothed, is substituted by a weighted average of the counts in the corresponding pixel of the preceding and succeeding frames as illustrated in Figure 8-9. The weighted-average pixel count is calculated using the following algorithm:

$$P_j(new) = W_{i-1} P_{i-1} + W_j P_j + W_{j+1} P_{j+1,}$$

where $P_j(new)$ is the weighted-average pixel count, P_j is the original number of counts in the pixel, P_{j-1} is the number of counts in the corresponding pixel in the preceding frame, while P_{j+1} is the number of counts in the corresponding pixel in the succeeding frame, while W_j, $W_{j-1,}$ and W_{j+1} are the weights applied to the respective pixels. Usually, the weighting coefficients are the same as the top

NUCLEAR CARDIOLOGY 161

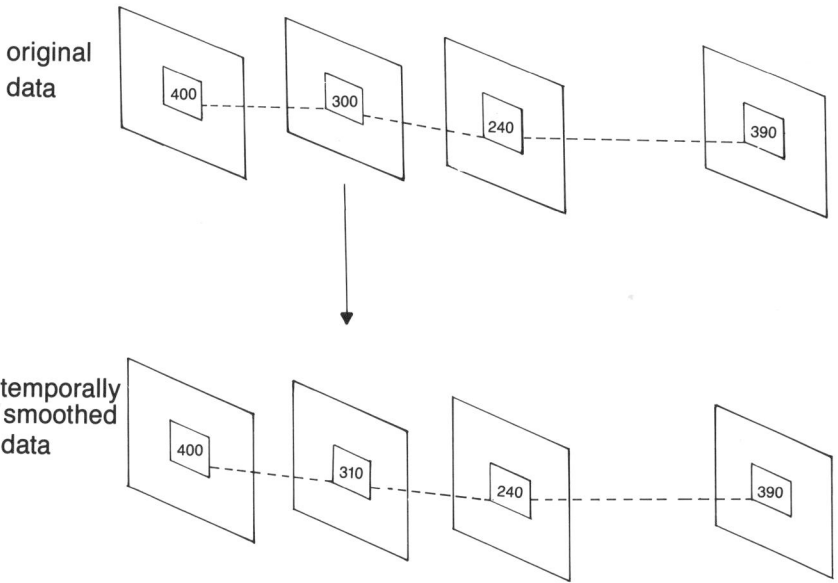

FIGURE 8-9 Temporal smoothing makes the counts in each pixel change gradually from frame to frame, resulting in less fluctuation of the volume curve and reduction of flickers during cine display.

row of coefficients in the nine-point smoothing kernel, i.e. $W_{j-1} = 1$, $W_j = 2$, $W_{j+1} = 1$. As a numerical example, suppose $P_{j-1} = 400$, $P_j = 300$, and $P_{j+1} = 240$. Upon applying the temporal smoothing algorithm to the data, we get,

$$P_j(\text{new}) = 1/4(400) + 1/2(300) + 1/4(240) = 310.$$

Because the first frame of the image series does not have a preceding frame, the pixel counts are averaged by taking a weighted average of the first and the second frames as follows:

$$P_j(\text{new}) = 3/4 \, P_1 + 1/4 \, P_2,$$

where P_1 and P_2 are the first and second frame in the multi-gated series, respectively.

The last frame of the image series is smoothed using a technique called *wrapped around,* which takes a weighted average of the counts in the corresponding pixels in the second to the last frame, the last frame, and the first frame of the series as follows:

$$P_{last}(\text{new}) = 1/4\ P_{last-1} + 1/2\ P_{last} + 1/4\ P_1,$$

where P_{last-1}, P_{last} and P_1 are counts in the corresponding pixels in the second to the last, the last, and the first frames, respectively. The assumption here is that the last and first frames in the series are actually two adjacent time intervals in the cardiac cycle. That is why the first frame in the series is treated like a succeeding frame in the smoothing process. The pixel counts in the first frame are not averaged by counts in the last frame, however. As previously discussed, the last several frames in the series invariably have a fewer number of counts due to errors resulting from fluctuations in the R-R time intervals. If we average the pixel counts in the first frame with the counts in the last frame, we would be erroneously reducing the number of counts in the first frame and adversely affecting the accuracy of the EF to be calculated later.

Frame Normalization

Ideally the last several frames in the series should have nearly the same number of counts as in the initial frames. Due to arrhythmic contractions, however, the acquisition time for the last several frames of the series is usually shorter than for those at the beginning, resulting in a loss of counts. To compensate for the loss of counts due to variations in the R-R time interval, we could make these frames to have the same number of counts by multiplying the number of counts in each pixel by a normalization factor. The normalization factor for a given frame is calculated as a ratio of the total number of counts in the first frame to the total number of counts in the frame to be corrected:

$$F = \frac{\text{Total number of counts in the first frame}}{\text{Total number of counts in a given frame}},$$

where F is the normalization factor. For frames that have the same number of counts as the first frame, the correction factor is 1. Those frames near the end of the cardiac cycle have a fewer number of counts and the correction factor is greater than 1. After normalization the last several frames in the series should have nearly the same number of counts as in the first frame.

This count normalization procedure does not distort the image pattern because every pixel is multiplied by the same factor. Hence, the contrast between the pixels remains the same. The normalization process is commonly used to reduce the amount of flickering during cine display. Normalization is helpful if the variation of the beat lengths is small. With large fluctuations in the R-R intervals, counts accumulated in a given time interval actually come from widely different phases of the cardiac cycle. Under such circumstances one of the bad-beat rejection techniques must be used at the time of acquisition.

After these preprocessing steps, heart wall motion can be assessed by studying the pulsating pattern of the smoothed and normalized blood-pool image in cine mode. The cyclical rate of the image frames is operator adjustable so that the motion of the blood pool can be studied at different display speeds. For computers with a large display memory, the monitor screen can be divided into 4-16 windows. Within each window a different series of multiple-gated images may be displayed in cine mode at the same time. These images can be acquired from the patient on different days or from different angles of projection. Studies have shown that such simultaneous visual assessment of the cine display is both a sensitive and an accurate method for detecting cardiac dysfunctions.

There is an alternate method to study the wall motion than displaying the blood-pool images in cine. The edge of the blood pool in the left ventricle can be outlined by one of the ROI methods to represent the ventricular wall. These ROIs are then displayed on the monitor in cine mode. Cinematic display of the contours has the advantage of allowing the observer to focus his attention on the edges of the moving blood pool. With this form of display, the outline of the ventricle in diastole is used as the frame of reference and remains stationary, while the ROIs corresponding to the other phases of the ventricular contraction are displayed in cine. Using the outline of the left ventricle in end-diastole (ED) as a position marker, the abnormal area of contraction can be more easily detected.

QUANTITATIVE DATA ANALYSES

Left ventricular ejection fraction (LVEF) is considered by cardiologists to be one of the most valuable prognostic and diagnostic indicators of cardiac pump function. Therefore, all software for multiple-gated blood-pool studies strive toward calculating this numerical index accurately, consistently, and rapidly. We can derive several other pertinent numerical indices, such as the peak ejection rate and the peak filling rate, from the same data used to calculate the EF. However, these parameters are not routinely calculated, but they are useful as adjunct information in the management of patients with heart disease.

The equilibrium blood-pool studies are based on the assumption that the activity seen by the gamma camera is directly proportional to the blood volume. Thus, changes of activity in a chamber of the heart, as seen by the gamma camera, are directly related to the blood volume changes in that chamber. This is one of the major advantages of gated blood-pool studies over contrast angiography, i.e., the blood volume changes can be measured without having to make any assumption on the geometric shape of the heart chamber.

Left Ventricular Regions of Interest

Outlining the left ventricle with a region of interest (ROI) accurately and consistently is the key to successful calculation of EF. Yet it is one of the most difficult tasks. For computation of the procedure requires drawing four ROIs, one ROI over the image of the left ventricle in ED, one end-diastolic background ROI, one ROI over the ventricle in ES, and one ROI for the background activity during ES. After the diastolic and systolic images have been corrected for the background activity (Bkg), the number of counts within each ventricular ROI is used to calculate the EF according to the formula:

$$F = \frac{(ED\ counts\ -\ ED\ Bkg)\ -\ (ES\ counts\ -\ ES\ Bkg)}{ED\ counts\ -\ ED\ Bkg}.$$

Drawing an ROI accurately and consistently over the left ventricle is difficult, especially during ES, where the image of the left ventricle becomes so small that it sometimes blends in with the aorta. Because of the tedium and subjectivity involved with hand-drawing the ROI, a number of computer methods, such as count thresholding and the first-and second-derivative algorithms, have been devised as a labor-saving and unbiased means to estimate ventricular edges. Although excellent correlation of the EFs with those calculated from radiographic techniques have been reported, the ventricular outlines and, hence the EF, are not always as faithfully reproduced by the computer as one may be led to believe by the computer enthusiast. The left ventricular edge can be consistently tracked by the computer if it has high count statistics and is well isolated from the other anatomic structures of the heart. The computer fails miserably if the statistical noise is high and if the contrast between the left ventricle and the rest of the structures in the image is low.

For images with poor count statistics, there will be large fluctuations in the activity profile. These fluctuations are amplified further by truncation errors and imprecisions in the computer calculation of the first and second derivatives. As a result, the computer-generated ROI can vary widely from one trial to the next. Manipulating the image with a smoothing filter can reduce some of the statistical noise, but this is done at the expense of reducing the contrast between the left ventricle and its surrounding structures.

In some studies ^{99m}Tc may be poorly tagged to the red blood cells. Hence, the ventricular blood-pool activity is not much greater than the free ^{99m}Tc activity in the background. Under such circumstances, the computer-generated ROIs tend to become oversized. With high background activities, the counts acquired into the computer images come mostly from the background structures and not from the left ventricle. Poor count statistics in the left ventricle coupled with high background activity often misleads the computer to draw rather bizzare-shaped regions. According to my personal bias, whenever the multiple-gated images are presented with poor ventricular counts and high background activity, a trained observer can define the ventricular borders more consistently and accurately than the computer.

The Volume Curve

The volume curve as illustrated in Figure 8-10 is also known as the time-activity curve. It is generated as a companion to the EF to show

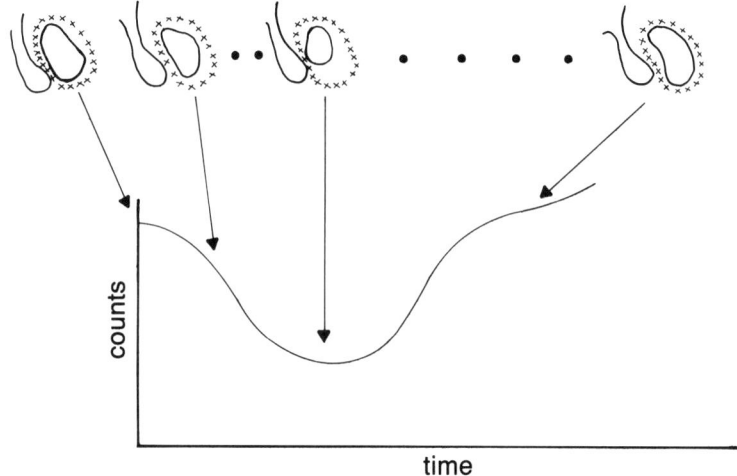

FIGURE 8-10 Counts within a fixed ROI over the left ventricle at different phases of the cardiac cycle were used to construct this volume curve.

the time course of blood volume changes in the left ventricle during an average cardiac cycle. There are two common methods to generate such a volume curve, the fixed ROI method and the variable ROI method. The fixed ROI method assumes that the background activity remains constant and equal to the value computed from the diastolic background ROI. The ROI drawn over the left ventricle at diastole is superimposed over each of the background subtracted images in the image series. The volume curve is constructed by plotting the number of counts within the ROI as a function of time. This fixed ROI method is the most rapid way of constructing the volume curve and contains less statistical fluctuations as the variable ROI method. However, it makes an implicit assumption that the background counts remain constant throughout the cardiac cycle and that the counts included within the diastolic ROI are those from the left ventricle only. These two assumptions may not necessarily be true for all patient studies.

The variable ROI method makes the assumption that the background and the ventricular count distributions may be different in every image. Therefore, a pair of ventricular and background ROIs is generated for each image in the series. The number of counts within each ventricular ROI is then computed after the image has been corrected for background activity using the corresponding background ROI. The variable ROI method is more time-consuming because of the extra time required to generate two ROIs for each image and the additional steps required to calculate the background counts. The variable ROI volume curve generally shows greater statistical fluctuations than one generated by a fixed ROI, due to the greater variability among the left ventricular and background ROIs used to compute the counts in the respective regions. The reason for using the variable ROI method is that a volume curve so generated is more representative of the actual volume changes for each phase of the cardiac cycle. Studies have shown that the EFs calculated from the variable ROI method yielded better correlation than the fixed ROI method with radiographic studies. Regardless of whether the volume curve is generated by the fixed or variable ROI method, a three-point and ocassionally a five-point smoothing kernel is applied to the resulting volume curve to reduce some of the statistical fluctuations.

Based on the volume curve, several numerical indices can be calculated. The three most prominent are EF, peak ejection rate, and peak filling rate. The peak ejection rate is the maximum negative slope of the volume curve, while the peak filling rate is the maximum positive slope. The peak ejection rate has been shown to bear a direct relationship with the peak systolic pressure, while the peak filling rate can be used as an indirect measurement of end-diastolic dilatation. Perhaps due to our uncertainty about the normal values for the peak ejection rate and the peak filling rate, these two parameters are utilized only occasionally for the assessment of the cardiac disorders.

Functional Images

Functional images are not generated for enhancing the spatial resolution of the original images, but to illustrate the relative count changes in each pixel as an aid in the evaluation of the heart function. The EF image is an example of a functional image and it is produced by applying the EF equation:

$$EF = \frac{\text{end-diastolic image - end-systolic image}}{\text{end-diastole image}} \times 100\%$$

to the end-diastolic and end-systolic images on a pixel-to-pixel basis. The EF for each pixel is then displayed in color code. The resulting EF image provides us a visual display of the spatial distribution of the EF.

The *stroke volume image,* as shown in Figure 8-11, is formed by subtracting the systolic image from the diastolic image. The resultant image, somewhat resembling a horseshoe, reflects the relative distribution of activity ejected from the ventricle during systole. Since the activity is directly proportional to the blood volume, the stroke volume image is a display of the relative distribution of blood ejected from the left ventricle during systole. The stroke volume can be used to quantify the absolute volume of blood ejected if the number of counts per unit volume is known. However, such a calibration factor is difficult to obtain accurately due to variable amounts of tissue attenuation. Thus, we should interpret the stroke volume image qualitatively as a map of the relative contribution of the different regions of the ventricle to the stroke volume rather than as the absolute volume change.

When the diastolic ROI is superimposed on the stroke volume image, the ROI along the free wall of the ventricle should align with the edge of the stroke volume. So if we overlay the diastolic ROI on top of the stroke volume image, we can easily detect edges that are drawn much too far outside or inside the ventricular walls. This simple quality assurance procedure for checking the accuracy of the diastolic ROI is especially handy for those images with high background activities.

To automatically calculate EF, radii are drawn from the geometric center of the stroke volume image as the initial step of the second-derivative method to define the ventricular ROI. This technique obviates the necessity for the operator to mark the rough center of the ventricle before the start of the edge detection routine. As the ROI is refined after each iteration, the center is gradually shifted toward the activity center of the ventricle.

The *parodox image* is a close cousin of the stroke volume image. It is produced by subtracting the diastolic image from the systolic image. In a normal heart there are more counts in the ventricle during diastole than in systole. When the diastolic image is subtracted from the systolic image, the paradox image will contain negative values in the normal region of the ventricles. In a dyskinetic region

NUCLEAR CARDIOLOGY

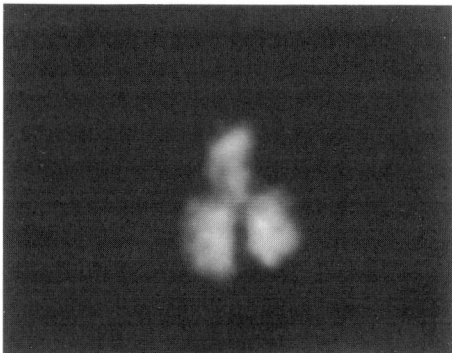

Diastolic Image

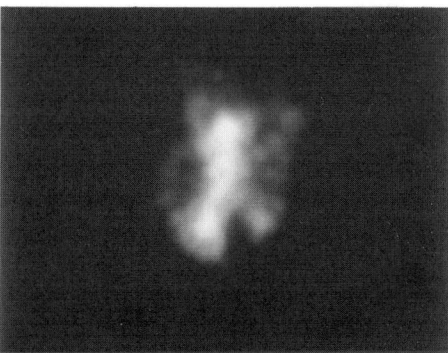

Systolic Image

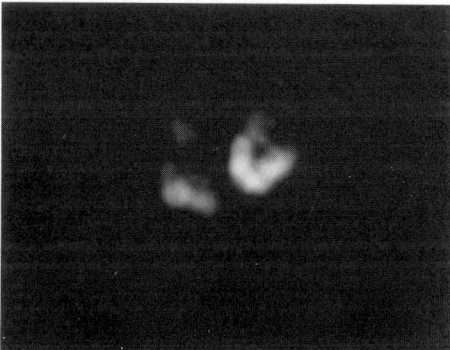

Stroke Volume Image

FIGURE 8-11 The stroke-volume image is obtained by subtracting the systolic image from the diastolic image.

of the free ventricular wall, however, the abnormal segment may bulge into the background region not previously occupied by the ventricles in diastole as shown in Figure 8-12. As a result, the dyskinetic segment will give rise to positive values in the paradox image. When the paradox image is shown, the normal regions will appear black because the negative values are converted to zeroes. The dyskinetic regions will appear in a shade of gray or color in proportion to the positive value in the pixel. In principle, the paradox image can reveal dyskinetic segments in the center as well as along the edge of the ventricles. In practice, the usefulness of the paradox image is confined to the assessment of the abnormalities in the free walls. Motion abnormalities lying perpendicular to the plane of the image are more suitably analyzed using the phase image.

Phase Analysis

The term *phase analysis* is confusing to people not familiar with Fourier mathematics. A technically inaccurate but more easily under-

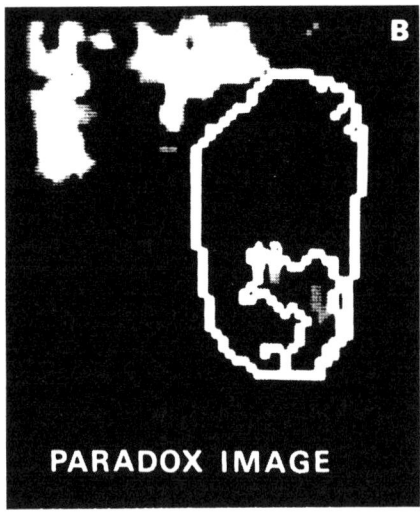

FIGURE 8-12 The paradox image is obtained by subtracting the diastolic image from the systolic image. (Reprinted with permission. Holman BL, et al. The paradox image: a noninvasive index of regional left ventricular dyskinesis. Figure 4. *J Nucl Med* 1979;20:1237-1242).

stood term for phase analysis is *rhythm analysis*. Phase analysis of multiple-gated cardiac images results in two images, the phase image and the amplitude image. The phase image is a graphic representation of the pulsatile synchronization of each heart segment, while the amplitude image measures the strength of the pulsatile motion and is, to a first-order approximation, proportional to the stroke volume.

Phase analysis treats each pixel as a small independent blood pool. Suppose a multiple-gated study is acquired as 24 frames of 64 x 64 images. We could arbitrarily select one pixel and plot a curve using the counts in the corresponding pixel in each of the 24 frames. The resulting curve is a one-pixel time-activity curve. If that pixel happens to fall within the boundary of the heart, the single-pixel time-activity curve represents the blood volume changes during the R-R interval in that one tiny segment of the heart. For a 64 x 64 image matrix, we could construct an activity-versus-time curve for each pixel and produce 4,096 of such time activity curves to describe the variation of activity in the camera field of view during an average R-R interval.

Phase analysis begins with performing a Fourier transform on each of the one-pixel time-activity curves. As explained in Chapter 6, Fourier analysis assumes that any periodic function, such as the ventricular time-activity curve, can be reconstructed using a sum of sine and cosine waves of different phases, amplitudes and frequencies. The current practice in cardiac phase analysis is to transform the time-activity curve to the frequency domain using only the first harmonic of a cosine wave, i.e., the fundamental frequency. The goodness of fit will improve by including the higher frequency terms (the higher order harmonics). For the purpose of calculating the parameters of interest in cardiac studies, however, the ventricular time-activity curve is adequately approximated by a sinusoidal function at the heart rate frequency. Besides, given the high statistical uncertainties associated with the limited number of counts in a single pixel, including the higher frequency terms in the Fourier transform only increases the computation time without affecting the final outcomes in most cases.

Fourier transform of the one-pixel time-activity curve yields two numerical indices, the amplitude and the phase angle. Basically, the amplitude defines the magnitude of contraction, while the phase angle defines the relative position of a pixel in the cardiac cycle to the other pixels. Two pixels are said to be in phase if their motions are perfectly synchronized. A brief explanation and example for calculating these two parameters for a simplified time-activity curve are presented in Appendix C.

Figure 8-13 shows the time-activity curves for a pixel in the left atrium and one in the left ventricle. The Fourier transform of these time-activity curves shows that the phase angle of the atrial time-activity curve deviates from that of the ventricular time-activity curve by 180°. In other words, the atrium is 180° out of step with the ventricle. Mathematically, when two sinusoidal curves are 180° out of phase with each other, one curve rises to the maximum at the time that the other curve is at its minimum. This phase rela-

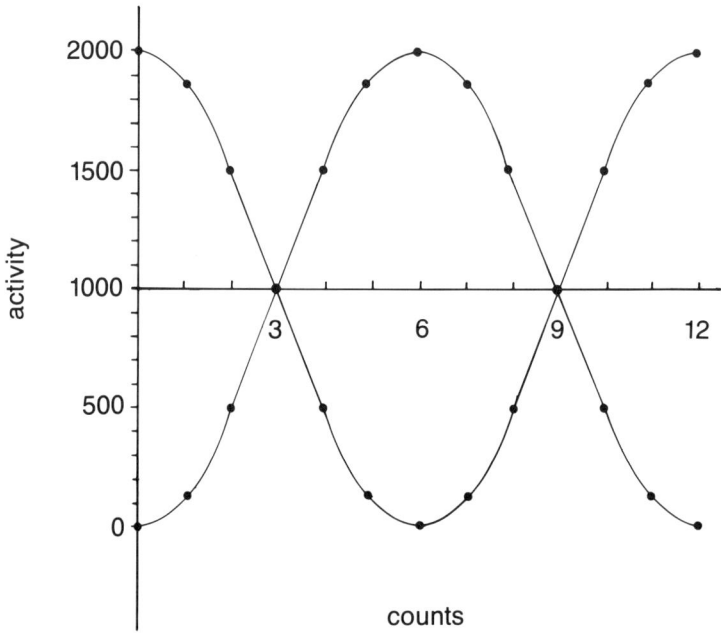

FIGURE 8-13 The atrium and ventricle are 180° out of phase because activity in the atrium is maximum while activity in the ventricle is at its minimum.

tionship between the atrium and ventricle corresponds well with the relative motion of these two chambers of the heart, (i.e., when the atrium is at its maximum contraction, the ventricle is at its maximum dilatation, and vice versa).

Presentation of Phase Analysis Results

If we arbitrarily assign a zero-degree phase angle to all pixels in the left and right ventricles at the onset of systole, then the phase angle of the pixels in the atria should be at 180°. However, the blood is not ejected instantaneously from every region of the atria or the ventricles. So, there is a distribution of phase angles within each chamber of the heart. A histogram plot of the phase angle of the pixels as shown in Figure 8-14 yields one peak centered around the 0° and another peak centered around 180°, corresponding to the phase angles of the atria and ventricles. The phase histogram is usually plotted in a continuum of colors with a designated color to represent

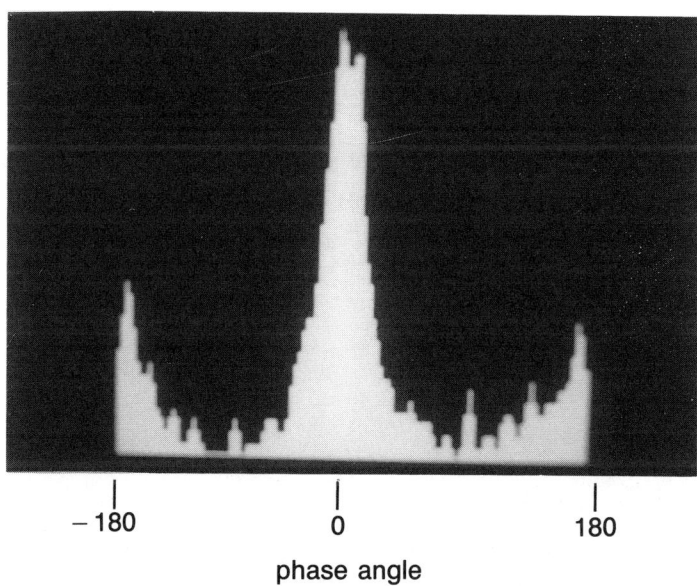

phase angle

FIGURE 8-14 When the phrase angles of all pixels within the heart are plotted, we obtain a histogram with two peaks. The peak near the 0° corresponds to the ventricles, and the 180° peak corresponds to the atria.

a given phase angle (Fig. 8-15). The color of each pixel in the phase image (the phase angle of that pixel) is assigned the same color as the corresponding phase angle in the histogram. Using this display format, the phase angle of a pixel can be inferred from the histogram.

Initial studies of the left ventricular phase histograms showed a sharp peak for normal individuals. For patients with abnormal ventricular wall functions, the phase histogram tends to yield a broader peak, meaning a greater spread of the phase angle distribution. In some studies of patients with aneurysm or left bundle block, the phase histogram often appears with two peaks. Unfortunately, extensive clinical trials failed to find a definitive correlation between the characteristics of the phase histogram with the functional defects of the ventricles.

In the phase image, the zero-degree phase angle is arbitrarily chosen to represent the onset of systole. This phase information is then used to study the electrical conduction pattern by blackening those pixels at each frame of the image series with a zero-degree phase angle. When the images are displayed in cinematic mode, the

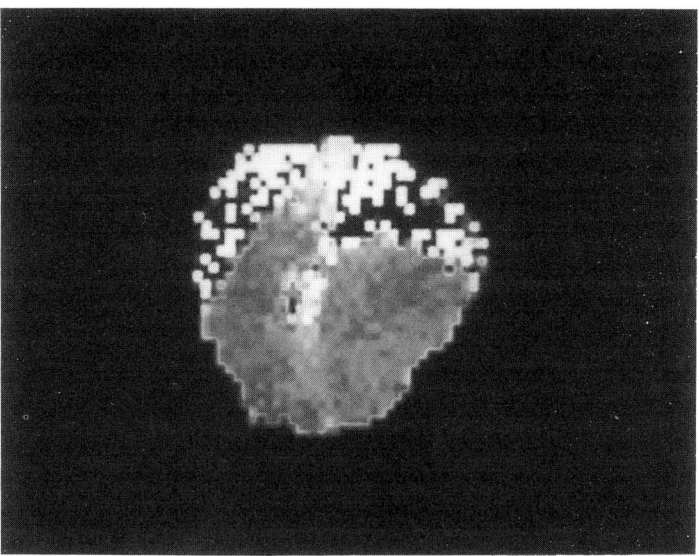

FIGURE 8-15 A phase image displays each pixel in a color corresponding to its phase angle. An abnormal region may appear in a color distinctly different from that of its neighbor.

blackened pixels appear as a wave of contraction propagating throughout the heart. In the normal heart, the contraction pattern is seen to originate from the atria and propagates down to the ventricles. Patients with pacemaker or conduction abnormalities produce a different electrical conduction pattern, and hence, an altered phase propagation pattern. Conceptually, we can study the wave propagation pattern of the phase images to assess various cardiac conduction disturbances. Unfortunately, there is insufficient patient data to firmly establish a guideline for correlating the phase pattern with various cardiac disturbances.

There is one application of the phase image not anticipated by the original investigators. In order to obtain an accurate EF, the ROI drawn around the left ventricle must not include any part of the left atrium. In many multiple gated studies, it is difficult to identify the valve plane that separates the left atrium from the left ventricle. Since the atria are filling when the ventricles are emptying, the phase image will show pixels in the atria 180° out of phase with those in the ventricles. Pixels in the region of the valve plane have a very different phase angle from that of the left atrium and ventricle and is shown in the phase image with a color distinctly different from these two chambers of the heart. Hence, the ROI can be traced through this distinctive color to isolate the ventricle from the atrium.

Amplitude Analysis

Each pixel in the amplitude image represents the magnitude of a one-pixel time-activity curve. Since counts are assumed to be proportional to the blood volume, the magnitude of change in the time-activity curve is assumed to be proportional to the change in blood volume under the pixel in the average cardiac cycle. The collection of these pixels in the amplitude image is, to a first approximation, proportional to the stroke volume image.

Unlike the stroke volume image obtained from subtracting the systolic image from the diastolic image, the amplitude image measures the total volume change regardless of when in the cardiac cycle that the change took place. In other words, the stroke volume image restricts the calculation of the count change between the diastolic and systolic frames, while the amplitude image calculates the maximum count difference without regard to which frames that the maximum and minimum points occur in the cardiac cycle. Hence, the amplitude image is not a true representation of the volume of blood ejected during systole. Proponents of amplitude analysis maintain that the stroke volume image may actually underestimate total volume change in a cardiac cycle because diastole and systole do not occur at the same time for all segments of the ventricle. Thus, the amplitude image is superior to the simple stroke volume image because it shows the actual volume of blood ejected from each region of the heart.

At the time of this writing, the amplitude image is not utilized for quantitative analyses. Instead, it is used in the same way as the stroke volume image by some investigators to assess the goodness of fit of the ROI over the ventricle and to form a mental picture of the regional distribution of count changes in a cardiac cycle. Many edge-detection programs also use the amplitude image as the seed or starting image to calculate the ROI for the left ventricle.

FIRST-PASS CARDIAC STUDIES

The first-pass technique is a complementary, and at times a competing, noninvasive technique with the multiple-gated method. For patients with severely irregular heart beats, the first-pass technique is preferred over the multiple-gated method for data acquisition because the data can be reformatted with great flexibility to form a representative set of images over a cardiac cycle. In addition, the first-pass method provides information not available with the multiple-gated equilibrium technique. For example, the right anterior oblique (RAO) view that the cardiologists traditionally used for contrast angiocardiography to visualize the anterior and inferior wall motions can be done only with the first-pass technique. The first-pass technique can be used to analyze the right and left ventricular functions as well as the pulmonary transit time functions. Furthermore, the acquisition time for a first-pass study takes more than 1 minute, while a multiple gated study typically takes 10 minutes to complete. However, first-pass studies have problems such as limited count statistics, few cardiac cycles for processing, and extra time required for reformatting of the data after acquisition.

Data Acquisition Technique

A common technique for dose administration involves injecting into the antecubital vein a highly concentrated bolus of 20 mCi ^{99m}Tc (in a volume > 0.5 ml), followed by 20 ml of saline flush. The saline flush accelerates the venous flow to the superior vena cava and reduces the diffusion of the tracer. Imaging is performed with the gamma camera oriented at the 30° RAO projection. Immediately following injection, counts are acquired into the computer for 30-45 seconds in either the list mode or the fast dynamic frame mode.

The high concentration of the bolus activity as it passes through the heart can produce a peak counting rate as high as 50,000 cps in a conventional single-crystal camera. With the older computers, such a fast stream of data must be acquired using the list mode in order to avoid missing an incoming count. The list mode technique records the (x, y) coordinates of each incoming count on the disk, or in the buffer memory sequentially as they arrive. List-mode acquisition, thus, requires a large buffer memory and disk storage to hold the data. The new generation of high speed computers with a large buffer memory, and high speed disk drives can acquire data in 64 x 64 dynamic frame mode as rapidly as 100 frames per second. Consequently, first-pass studies can be performed using these computers in rapid dynamic frame mode with excellent temporal resolution and very little count loss.

After acquisition, a simple quality assurance test should be performed to test the compactness of the injected bolus. The data are first reformatted from either the list mode or fast frame mode data, to 0.5 seconds per image. The series of 0.5-second images allows the operator to visualize the location of the superior vena cava. A time-activity curve is then constructed using a small ROI, usually a 4 x 4 square for a 64 x 64 image array, drawn over the superior vena cava. The bolus is acceptable if the full width at half maximum (FWHM) of the time-activity curve is less than 5 seconds. Data yielding a double-humped time-activity curve or a FWHM greater than 5 seconds are considered unsuitable for further analyses. The critical dependence on the injection technique is one of the weaknesses of the first-pass method.

METHODS OF DATA REFORMATTING FOR FIRST-PASS STUDIES

Unlike the multiple gated equilibrium studies, first-pass images need to be reformatted from the list-mode data or the rapid dynamic frames before it can be utilized to evaluate cardiac or pulmonary functions. Reformatting of the data for pulmonary function studies is straightforward, but there are several ways to format the data for ventricular function studies, depending on the types of information gathered and the method used to acquired the information.

Reformatting of ECG Gated List Mode Data

If the counts were acquired in list mode with both the time markers and R-wave triggers recorded, then the counts recorded during the passage of the bolus through the left ventricle can be sorted according to each R-R interval into the number of frames desired for one composite cardiac cycle, much like the series of images acquired from equilibrium gated studies. The first step in reformatting the data is to bracket the time interval that the bolus passes through the left ventricle. This is done by reformatting the original data into a series of 1-second frames. From the series of one-second frames, the operator can select the frames that the bolus starts appearing in and fading from the left ventricle. These two frame numbers then correspond to the time of the appearance and exiting of the bolus through the left ventricle. For most patients between 5 to 15 cardiac cycles are included in this time interval.

Next the operator selects the range of R-R time intervals acceptable for image reformatting, which is determined from the histogram of the R-R time intervals recorded throughout the duration of the list-mode acquisition. Usually, the range of R-R time values between the FWHM of the histogram are selected as the minimum and maximum beat length useful for data reformatting. Data collected in R-R intervals outside this selected range are rejected. Finally the acceptable beat length is divided into a number of time segments corresponding to the number of frames of images desired in a cardiac cycle. The duration of each frame in a given R-R interval is either stretched or compressed so that the same number of images are fit into each cardiac cycle. The final step in the reformatting process involves sorting the counts within each time segment into the respective frames of the series of images.

Reformatting of Non-ECG Gated List Mode Data

If the counts were aquired in list mode without the ECG trace, the data are reformatted using a *software gate* to sort the data into a series of composite images to represent an average cardiac cycle. The list-mode data are initially reformatted into a series of 1-sec frames. From this series of 1-second images, the frame that best shows the left ventricle is selected for a rough ROI to be drawn around it, taking care that no part of the right ventricle is included in the ROI. Also the time of the first appearance and the exiting of the activity in the ventricle is noted from the 1-second images. The list-mode data are reframed again starting from the time of the first appearance of the activity in the left ventricle to the time of the bolus exiting with a time per frame as short as one-tenth of a second in order to obtain good temporal resolution. A time-activity curve is next constructed using the ventricular ROI superimposed on these short duration images. The peaks and valleys in the time-activity curve as shown in Figure 8-16 are attributed to the blood volume changes in the left ventricle during diastole and systole, respectively. Normally data in 4-6 cardiac cycles with approximately equal peak-to-peak distance in the down-slope of the time-activity curve are selected for final reformatting. Suppose you want to form 16 composite images per cardiac cycle. The time interval between two adjacent peaks is divided into 16 equal segments. Counts in each of these time segments are then sorted into the corresponding image matrix to form a sequence of 16 composite images, (i.e., all counts collected in the first time segment following the activity peak are stored in Frame 1, counts occurring in the second time segment are put into Frame 2, and so on). The sequence is repeated with the second peak until data in all the selected cardiac cycles have been reformatted. Because only 4-6 cycles worth of data are used to form the composite images, the image noise is much higher than that in the multiple-gated images.

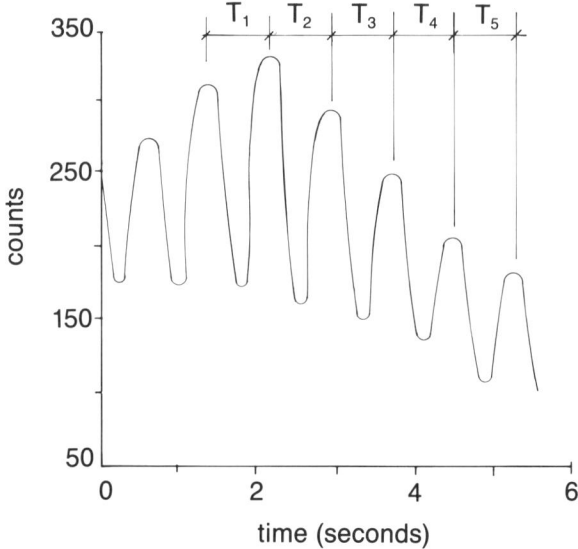

FIGURE 8-16 Images of list mode studies are reformatted from data in five to six cardiac cycles of nearly the same peak-to-peak distance on the time-activity curve of the injected bolus.

Reformatting of Rapid Dynamic Frames

The procedure for reformatting first-pass data from rapid dynamic frames is similar to reformatting from list-mode data by software gating. The difference is that they are already in the image frames. In order to draw a ventricular ROI, several of these fast dynamic frames are usually added together to increase the count statistics and thus the image resolution. This is one of the biggest advantages of dynamic frame acquisition for first-pass studies, adding image frames together takes much less time than reformatting from data in list mode.

A time-activity curve is then constructed by plotting the number of counts enclosed within the ROI in each frame as a function of time. Again, data in 4-6 heart beats with nearly equal peak-to-peak distance on the time-activity curve are selected for image reformatting. Each accepted R-R interval is divided into a number of segments corresponding to the number of frames desired in an average cardiac cycle. A set of composite images is formed by combining all those dynamic frames within each corresponding time segment of the selected beats to a series of composite images as shown in Figure 8-17. Since an acquisition rate in excess of 50 frames per second is easily achieved on computers with several megabytes of acquisition memory or high-speed disk drives, the temporal resolution of the composite image sequence is indistinguishable from the list mode data.

Ventricular Function Evaluations

Once the first-pass data have been reformatted to a series of composite images, we can evaluate many of the cardiac functions, such as the the EFs, ventrical size and wall motion, using the same techniques devised for multiple-gated studies. Although the count statistics of the first-pass images obtained with a gamma camera are poor, the calculated LVEFs correlate well with the results from multiple-gated studies and contrast angiography.

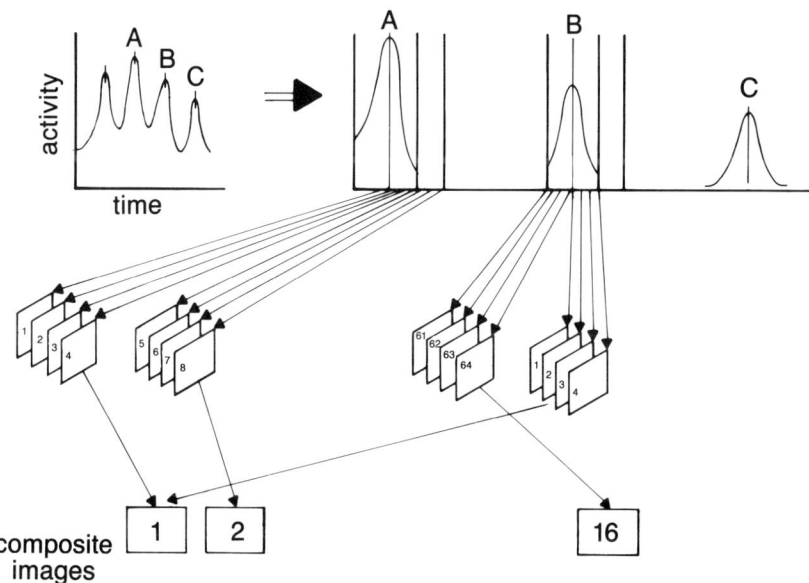

FIGURE 8-17 First-pass studies are currently done using the rapid dynamic frame acquisition method. Frames from the same phase of different cycles are added together to form a series of composite images.

Conceptually, the first-pass technique is the technque of choice for calculating the RVEF because the activity in the right ventricle can be temporally separated from those in the left ventricle, (i.e., only those counts collected during the time that the bolus passes through the right ventricle are selected for image reformatting). Due to difficulty with angulating the gamma camera toward the patient and overlapping of activity in the right atrium, separation of the right ventricular border from its outflow tract is difficult in many patients.

The first-pass technique is not suitable for sequential measurement of the EF under graded exercises. Concern for the radiation dose to the patient from repeat injections is one of the prime reasons. Activities left over from the previous injection will not only reduce the image contrast to make drawing of the ventricular ROI difficult, but the high level of background activity will also interfere with accurate calculation of the activities within the ventricular ROI from the second injection. If sequential first-pass studies are to be performed using ^{99m}Tc as the tracer, we commonly have to wait one to two hours for the background activity to reduce before commencing with the repeat study. Gold-195m with a half-life of 30 seconds has been used to overcome the problems of radiation dose and residual background activities. Unfortunately, the ^{195m}Au/^{195m}Hg generator is expensive and is not readily available. Also, in order to take advantage of the short-lived ^{195m}Au as the tracer, the gamma camera must be able to handle in excess of 100,000 cps without a severe degradation of resolution. This requirement will preclude the use of all but the latest generation of gamma cameras and multi-crystal cameras.

Detection of Intra-cardiac Shunts

Both right-to-left and left-to-right shunts can be detected and quantified using the first-pass technique. The detection of left-to-right shunts is performed by comparing the pulmonary blood flow with the systemic flow. The right-to-left shunts, on the other hand, are detected by early appearance of activity in the left ventricle and the use of a different radiopharmaceutical.

Left-to-right shunt studies are performed by measuring the transient flow characteristics of the tracer through the lungs using the first pass technique. With the gamma camera positioned anterior to the lungs, counts are collected either in list mode or in dynamic frame mode with a framing rate from one to four frames per second for 30 seconds, depending on the patient's heart rate. If counts are acquired in list mode, they are reformatted from 0.25 seconds to 1 second per frame. Next, a ROI is drawn over the lungs to construct a time-activity curve (Fig. 8-18) to characterize the transient pulmonary blood flow.

Under normal blood circulation, the ratio of the tracer flow through the lungs versus the flow through the systemic circulation equals 1. With a left-to-right shunt, the tracer returns to the lungs without first going through the systemic circulation. Early return of the tracer to the lungs, thus, makes the pulmonary versus systemic flow ratio greater than one.

The next step in quantifying the pulmonary-to-systemic flow ratio is by fitting the major peak in the lung activity curve to a gamma variate function as shown in Figure 8-18. The gamma variate func-

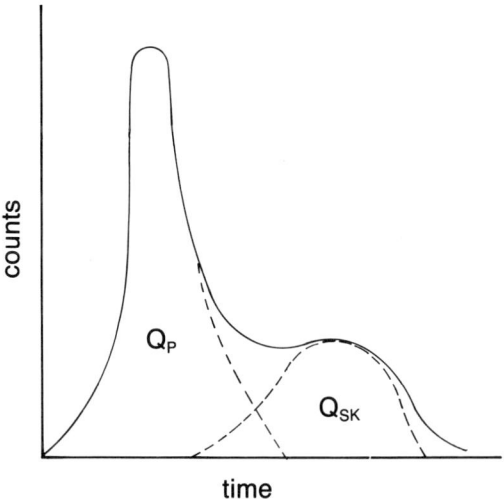

FIGURE 8-18 The time-activity curve of the bolus as it passes through the lungs is characterized by two gamma functions. Area under the first and second gamma functions (Q_p and Q_s) are proportional to the pulmonary and systemic flows, respectively. Left-to-right shunt is indicated if the ration of Q_p/Q_s is greater than 1.3.

tion is an exponential function similar to the familiar Gaussian function. Unlike the symmetrical bell-shaped Gaussian function, the gamma function is non-symmetrical and skews toward the origin. The pulmonary blood flow is assumed to be proportional to the quantity, Q_p, which is calculated as the area under the fitted gamma variate function.

The fitted gamma function, representing the pulmonary blood flow, is then subtracted from the original lung-activity curve to make the early recirculation peak stand out. The recirculation peak, if any, represents the shunt portion of the pulmonary blood flow curve. The recirculation peak is fitted with another gamma function and the area under the second fitted curve is calculated to obtain the quantity Q_{sh}. The area under the second gamma function Q_{sh} represents the quantity of blood bypassed the systemic flow and returned prematurely to the pulmonary flow through the shunt.

The difference between the pulmonary flow Q_p and the amount recirculated through the shunt Q_{sh} is then equal to the systemic flow Qsh, i.e.,

$$Q_s = Q_p - Q_{sh}$$

The ratio of pulmonary flow-to-systemic flow is the Q_p/Q_{sh} ratio:

$$Q_p/Q_{sh} = Q_p / (Q_p - Q_{sh})$$

In the absence of left-to-right shunt, Q_{sh} is equal to zero and the ratio would be equal to 1. Through extensive patient studies, shunt is indicated whenever the Q_p/Q_{sh} ratio is greater than 1.3.

The major difficulty with the gamma variate method to quantify shunts is the statistical fluctuation of the curve data. Random noise in the lung-activity curve may cause the computer to derive a poorly fitted gamma function to the lung-activity curve.

A right-to-left shunt can be determined by comparing the time course of the bolus activity passing through the left and right ventricles and the lungs. In the presence of a right-to-left shunt, some of the activity goes directly into the left ventricle without first passing through the lungs. As a result, there will be an early peak in the left ventricular activity curve appearing at approximately the same time with the peak in the time-activity curve of the right ventricle and ahead of the lung-activity peak as shown in Figure 8-19.

PLANAR QUANTIFICATION OF MYOCARDIAL PERFUSION

As an analog of potassium, ^{201}Tl is extracted by the myocardial cells in proportion to the amount of regional blood flow. Thus, regions of myocardial infarction and stress-induced ischemia with reduced blood flow can be detected as cold spots in ^{201}Tl images. Ischemic areas appear as perfusion defects in the thallium image at peak exercise, but the defects disappear partially or completely after redistribution at rest.

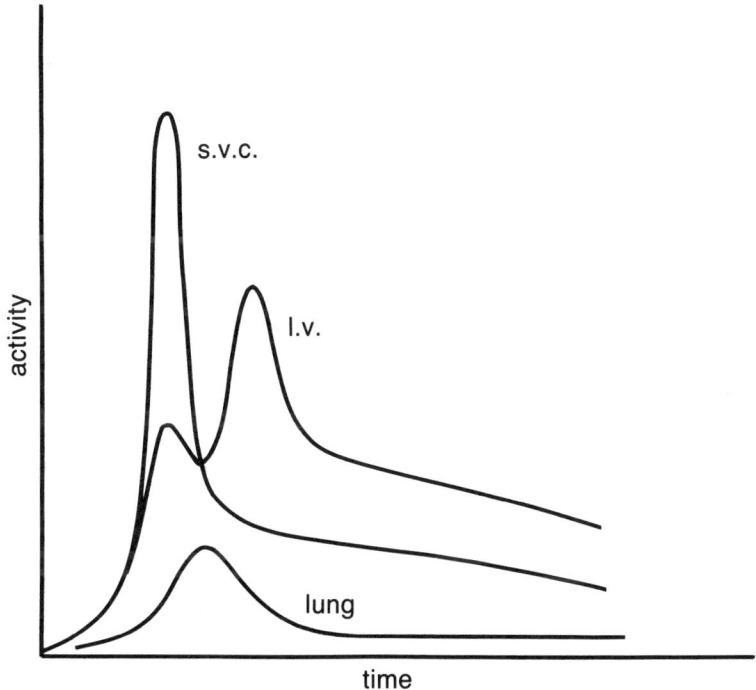

FIGURE 8-19 Arrival of tracer in the left ventricle at about the same time it arrives in the lungs is indicative of right-to-left shunt.

Interpretation of the thallium perfusion images based on visual perception alone is difficult because the defects often show up as small regions in the image with subtle reduction in the count density. Compounding the difficulty with the image interpretation is that the observer has to make subjective assessment of the relative count density changes in images taken at rest and after stress. As an attempt to increase the sensitivity and objectivity with detecting ischemic defects, several methods have been devised, utilizing the computer to detect and quantify possible areas of ischemia. Although there are differences among the various thallium quantification algorithms, the essence of all the procedures is similar and can be summarized as follows.

Prior to the quantification step, the images are processed using the interpolative background subtraction method to increase the contrast and smoothed spatially to suppress the random noise. By means of a light pen or other pointing devices, the operator makes a mark at the center of the ventricle. The computer then draws a number of radii from this point and out to the background area. Depending on the software used, these radii are layed out from 2° to 9° apart and spans 360° around the entire heart. Next, the computer searches for the pixel with the maximum number of counts along each radius. The resulting plot of the maximum pixel counts in each radius (Fig. 8-20) is commonly known as the circumferential profile. From this activity profile, the perfusion of thallium in one myocardial segment is compared with that of another, hence, informing us of the relative amount of blood flow.

The thallium quantification procedure is always applied to a pair of images taken immediately after peak exercise and after a 4-hour or 24-hour resting period. The idea is that perfusion defects seen in the ischemic areas immediately after exercise may return to normal after a resting period. By superimposing the circumferential profiles of the stress and delayed image in the same plot, the observer can readily identify the ischemic regions. In addition to intercomparison of the patient's own circumferential profiles at stress and after resting, the profiles can be compared with the distribution patterns of the normal population, thereby reducing the chance false-positive interpretations.

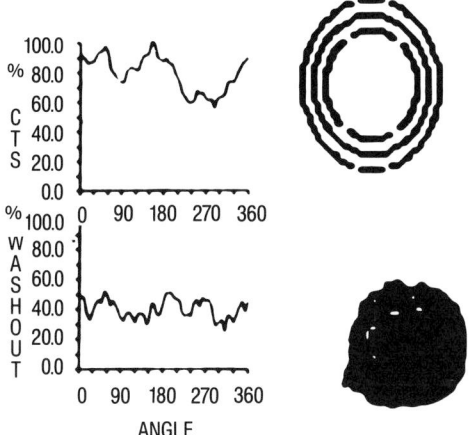

FIGURE 8-20 Perfusion of a ^{201}Tl in the myocardium is characterized quantitatively by tracing a circumference of maximum pixel activity (Reprinted with permission. Joseph Areeda, et al. Improved analysis of thallium-201 myocardial scintigrams: Quantitation of distribution, washout, and redistribution. (Reprinted with permission from Esser P, ed. *Digital imaging.* New York: The Society of Nuclear Medicine; 1982:257-269).

CONCLUSION

Many elegant computer methods have been developed in the past decade to meet the clinical needs for accurate and consistent quantitative results. It is hoped that this simplified explanation of the physical principles and their implementation on the computer has helped to remove the mystery surrounding image acquisition and processing procedures. Manufacturers of nuclear medicine computers also devote much of their resources towards optimizing their hardware and software for the demanding nuclear cardiac studies. Therefore, readers who are interested in learning the intricacies of computer image processing will find it rewarding to study the algorithms and program structures used in their cardiac software package.

SUGGESTED READINGS

1. Bacharach SL, Green MV, Borer JS. Instrumentation and data processing in cardiovascular nuclear medicine: evaluation of ventricular function. *Semin Nucl Med* 1979;9:257-274.

2. Collins SM, Fleagle SR, Skorton DJ. Digital image processing fundamentals: application to cardiac imaging. *Am J Cardiac Imaging* 1987;1:3-17.

3. Green MV, Bacharac SL. Functional imaging of the heart: methods, limitations, and examples from gated blood-pool scintigraphy. *Prog Cardiovas Dis* 1986;28:319-348.

4. Reiber JHC. Quantitative analysis of left ventricular function from equilibrium gate blood-pool scintigrams: an overview of computer methods. *Eur J Nucl Med* 1985;10:97-110.

5. Holman BL, Wynne J, Iodine J, Zielonka J, Neill J. The paradox image: a noninvasive index of regional left ventricular dyskinesis. *J Nucl Med* 1979;19:1237-1242.

6. Wei C, Henkin RE, Hale DJ, Hall D. Methods for detection of left ventricular edges. *Semin Nucl Med* 1980;10:39-53.

7. Wendt RE, Murphy PH, Clark JW, Burdine JA. Interpretation of multigated Fourier function images. *J Nucl Med* 1982;23:715-724.

CHAPTER

9

SINGLE-PHOTON EMISSION COMPUTED TOMOGRAPHY

INTRODUCTION

Single-photon emission computed tomography (SPECT) is a radionuclide imaging technique which produces a picture of the radionuclide distribution within a thin section of the patient. A major advantage of SPECT is its ability to show radionuclide distribution in any slice of the body-coronal, sagittal, transverse, or oblique plane. This feature is of great value for detecting and accurately locating lesions in a complex anatomical structure. In addition to providing isolated view planes, SPECT yields a higher image contrast when compared with planar images because activities lying outside the plane of interest are reduced. Because SPECT can isolate activity in any plane within the body, it offers the potential for quantitative analyses that are difficult to do with the planar images.

In this chapter, a general description of a typical SPECT system and the technical considerations used to acquire and process the data to produce the tomographic images are presented. Emphasis will be placed on the role of computer methods in SPECT, data acquisition, quality assurance performance testing, and generating transverse images. Recognizing that learning the mathematical foundation of image reconstruction is essential for gaining an insight into the practical aspects of SPECT, an intuitive explanation of image reconstruction with the filtered backprojection algorithm is briefly discussed in the chapter.

INSTRUMENTATION—SYSTEM DESCRIPTION

A SPECT system consists of two basic components—a radiation detection device for measuring the radioactivity profiles at various angles around the patient, and a computer for processing the projection profiles to form an image of the cross-section.

Two general designs have been used to construct the radiation detection portion of the SPECT system. One approach utilizes several linear arrays of NaI detectors that rotate around the patient as illustrated in Figure 9-1. The other approach as shown in Figure 9-2 mounts a conventional gamma camera on a gantry that rotates around the patient to obtain projection profiles.

The scanner-based detectors collect projection profiles for one slice from several angles simultaneously, while the gamma camera-based detectors collect a number of projection profiles simultaneously at each angle of rotation. With a multiple number of detectors collecting counts around the patient simultaneously, the scanner-based SPECT system can complete its data acquisition in 10 minutes or less. Therefore, the scanner-based designs are more suitable than the camera-based designs for dynamic studies.

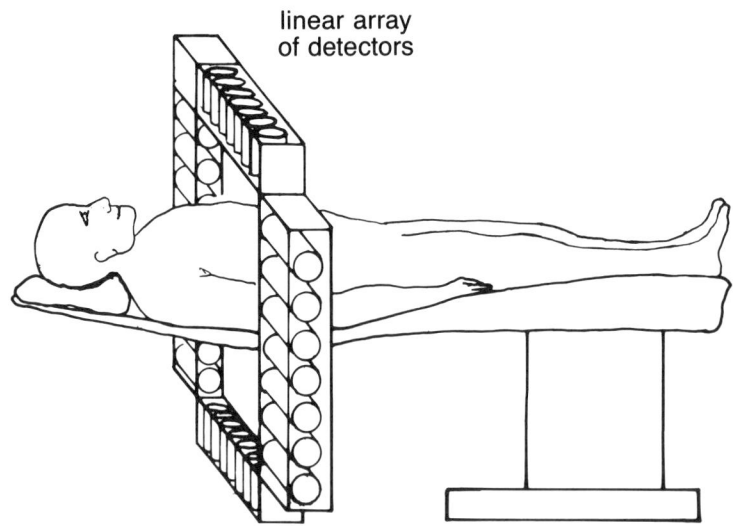

FIGURE 9-1 A dedicated SPECT system that uses four linear arrays of radiation detectors around the patient to gather projection data.

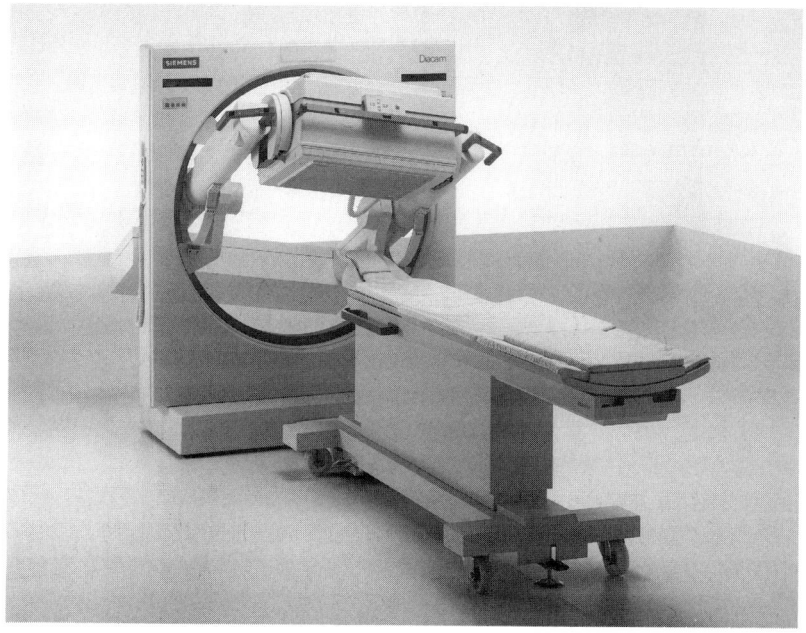

FIGURE 9-2 Most SPECT systems use a conventional gamma camera to rotate around the patient to acquire the projection data.

A camera-based SPECT system consists of a wide-field gamma camera mounted on a gantry, a patient support couch, and a computer as shown in Figure 9-2. The gantry is controlled by the computer to rotate around the patient according to a predefined pattern. Although some systems can acquire data with the detector in continuous motion, most systems use the step-and-shoot technique, in which the camera moves in stepwise rotation; image acquisition is done with the camera stopped at regular angular intervals around the patient. With image acquisition done one angle at a time, about 30 minutes are required to acquire one complete set of projection data for reconstruction. Hence, the camera-SPECT system is useful for static studies only. Because the camera-based detectors measure a number of contiguous slices simultaneously, tomographic images in the coronal, sagittal and oblique views can be more easily reconstructed than with a scanner-based detector. In addition, the SPECT system could use the gamma camera for planar imaging when not performing tomography. Due to this versatility and lower equipment cost, the gamma camera-based design is widely used on commercial SPECT systems.

The Computer System

Most of the computers used for the acquisition and processing of radionuclide images can be used to perform SPECT studies. One additional function that the computer in a SPECT system needs to do is control the rotation of the gantry. In order to obtain accurate reconstructed images, the gamma camera needs to acquire images at precise angular positions around the patient. The computer can handle this task easily by triggering the gantry at regular time intervals to rotate for a precise angular increment.

It is desirable that computers used for SPECT have a large central processing unit (CPU) or buffer memory and ample disk storage. This requirement is obvious if we consider that a typical SPECT study may have up to 180 projection images and 60 reconstructed images in each of the transverse, coronal, and sagittal planes. If the images were recorded in 64 x 64 word matrices, 3 MB of disk space will be needed to hold 360 images; if the images were acquired in 128 x 128 format, 12 MB wil be needed. Hence, the computer should have disk drives with 80 MB or greater capacity so that the most recent studies can be stored on-line for rapid retrieval. A system having a large CPU and/or buffer memory is desirable not only because it is needed for computations involving large image matrices, but also because it permits much of the intermediate calculation results to be kept in memory instead of having them shuttled back and forth between the disk and the memory. Since it takes much more time to access data stored on the disk than in the CPU memory, time spent in transferring data between the disk and the CPU memory can significantly increase the processing time. Thus, a large CPU or buffer memory will reduce much of this unnecessary data swapping and increases the overall processing speed.

Image reconstruction requires repetitive calculations on a large amount of projection data. An arithmetic operation, say addition or multiplication, can be done much more rapidly by a dedicated hardware device than by the CPU using software. For this reason, a hardware arithmetic device called the array processor is commonly added to the computer to increase its number crunching speed. Array processors are hardware devices designed to do only a limited variety of arithmetic operations on matrices and highly ordered array of numbers. However, their execution speed can be 100,000 times faster than the CPU using software alone. As an example, a 64 x 64 transaxial image may take nearly 1 minute to recontruct without an array processor; with the aid of an array processor, the time can be cut to less than 1 second.

One type of array processors achieves this high computation speed by delegating two or more microprocessors to carry out the arithmetic operations simultaneously. As described in Chapter 1, we call the process that breaks down an operation into several smaller steps to be carried out concurrently is called parallel or pipeline processing. To help the user achieve the maximum computation speed, the manufacturers of array processors usually supply a software package tailored to its special hardware design for the user to incorporate into their application programs. The typical arithmetic routines supplied by the manufacturer include fast Fourier transform and matrix multiplication and division. However, with the high-speed CPUs currently available, the service of an array processor is not as critical. Also, the speed performance of recent nuclear medicine computer systems based on the RISC architecture (discussed in Chapter 1) indicate that the days of array processors are numbered.

MATHEMATICS OF TRANSVERSE IMAGE RECONSTRUCTION

Virtually all commercial SPECT systems utilize the filtered backprojection method to reconstruct transverse images from the projection data. The theory of filtered backprojection algorithm is not explained in much detail here because it requires mathematics well beyond the scope of this primer. Instead, an empirical approach is used to show the essence of the filtered backprojection method without invoking heavy-duty mathematics.

The Simple Backprojection Method

Suppose we take an image of a point source with a gamma camera from three different angles, as in Figure 9-3. We next divide each

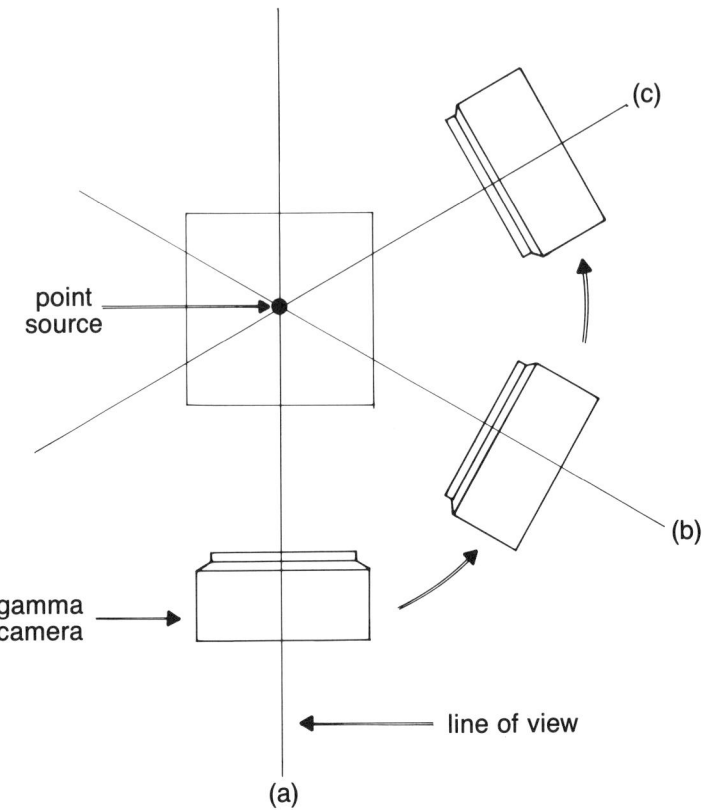

FIGURE 9-3 The projection profiles of the point source are obtained using the step-and-shoot technique. The gamma camera stops its rotation at regular angular increments to take images of the point source.

of these images into a number of strips and select the strip that passes through the image of the point source. If we plot the number of counts in each of the pixels across the selected strip, we obtain an activity profile as shown in Figure 9-4. The number of counts at each point in the projection profile is called the ray-sum because it represents the total number of counts seen by the gamma camera along a line of view, i.e., a ray.

Next, we hand these three projection profiles to a "whiz kid" and ask him to reconstruct the image of the point source on the computer. This is no problem for him since he has decided that the eas-

SPECT

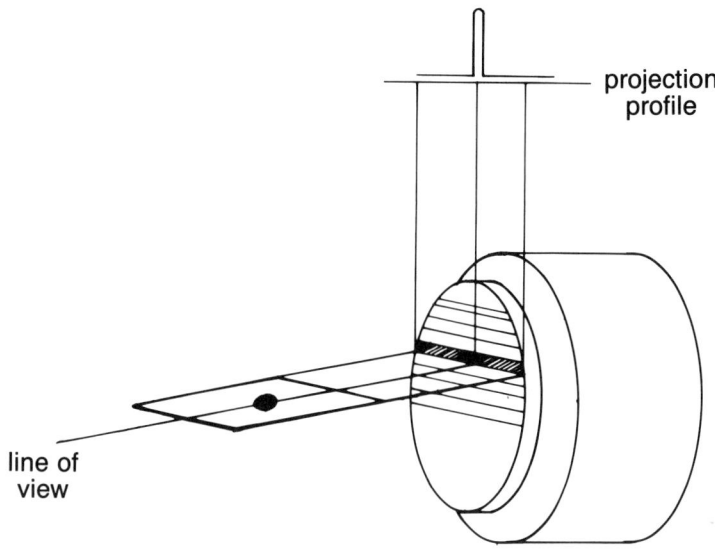

FIGURE 9-4 An activity profile is constructed by plotting the number of counts in the row of pixels that passes through the point source.

iest way is simply to cast the ray-sums from each of the three projection profiles into an image matrix in the computer. However, a ray-sum has no information on how the counts were distributed along the line of view of the gamma camera. He assumes that the counts in each ray-sum were distributed evenly among the pixels that lie along the path of the ray as shown in Figure 9-5A. Likewise, he projects the ray-sums from the second projection profile into the image plane and adds the counts together at the intersection of the two profiles (Fig. 9-5B). After superimposing all the ray-sums of the three projection profiles in the image plane, he reconstructs a transverse image of the point source (Fig. 9-5C). This method is known as simple backprojection.

The main advantage of simple backprojection is the ease with which we can construct a transverse tomogram without complicated mathematics or even a computer. The serious drawback of the simple backprojection technique is the starburst artifact in the reconstructed image in Figure 9-5C. The starburst artifact is especially prominent in an image containing a highly localized activity such as the point source in the example. We can somewhat blur the star-

A

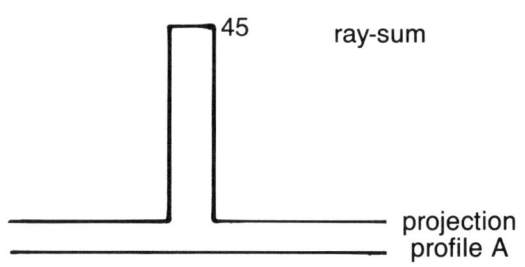

image plane

45 ray-sum

projection profile A

B

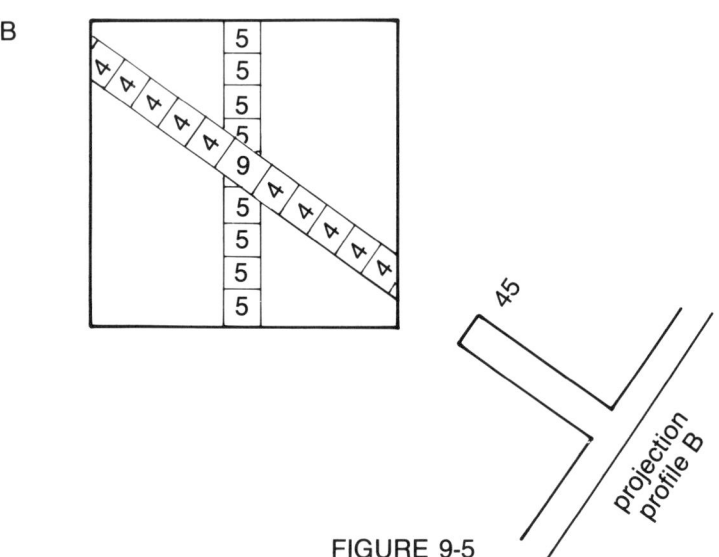

45

projection profile B

FIGURE 9-5

SPECT

C

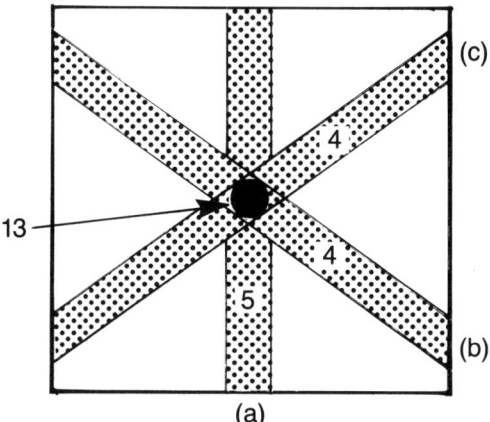

FIGURE 9-5 The simple backprojection method reconstructs an image by spreading each ray-sum evenly among the pixels along the projection line in the image plane.

burst artifacts by acquiring many projection profiles; but the image contrast is reduced because of the high background density.

The Filtered Backprojection Method

Because everybody made fun of him for producing such an esoteric image by simply dispersing the original activity profiles into the image plane, the "mathematical genius" decided to do some fudging on the original data before backprojection in order to get rid of those unsightly streaks in the reconstructed image. He modified each of the original projection profiles with a number scheme to produce a projection profile with a negative lobe on each side of the peak (Fig. 9-6). Given that there are no such things as negative counts in the real world measurements, let us see what the resulting image will look like after backprojecting these modified projection profiles with negative side lobes into the image plane.

In Figure 9-7, he again evenly distributed the counts in each ray-sum, negative and positive, in the nine pixels along the projection line in the image plane. In Figure 9-8, the ray-sums in the second modified projection profile were also projected equally into the pixels along each ray and added to the the count contributions from

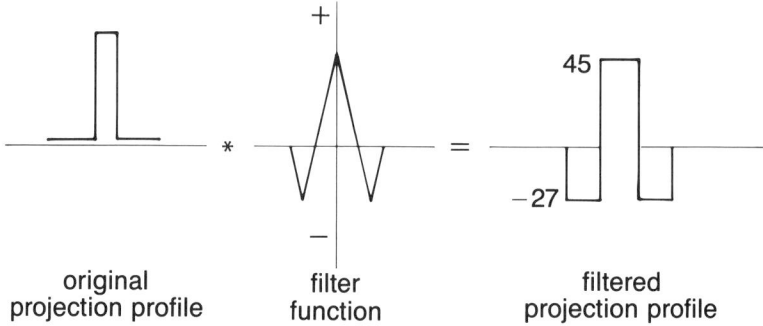

FIGURE 9-6 The filtered backprojection method modifies the original projection profile with a filter function before projecting the ray-sums into the image plane.

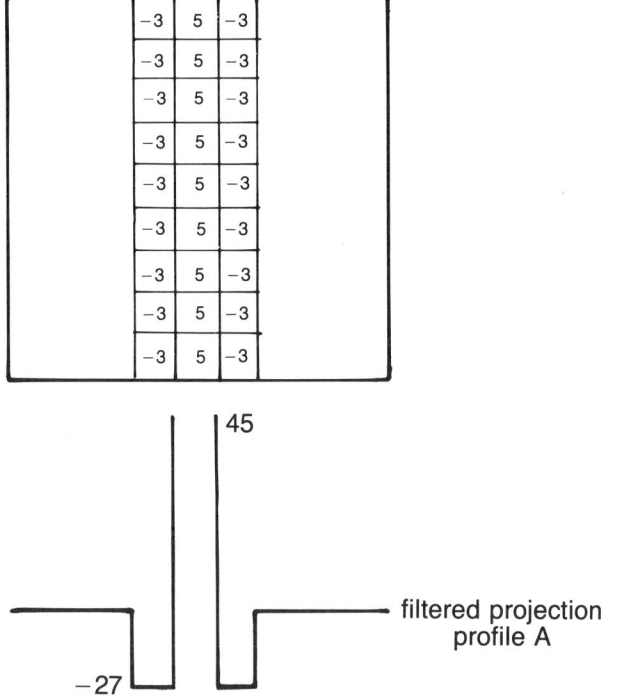

FIGURE 9-7 The positive and negative ray-sums in the first projection profile are evenly distributed in pixels along the projection lines in the image plane.

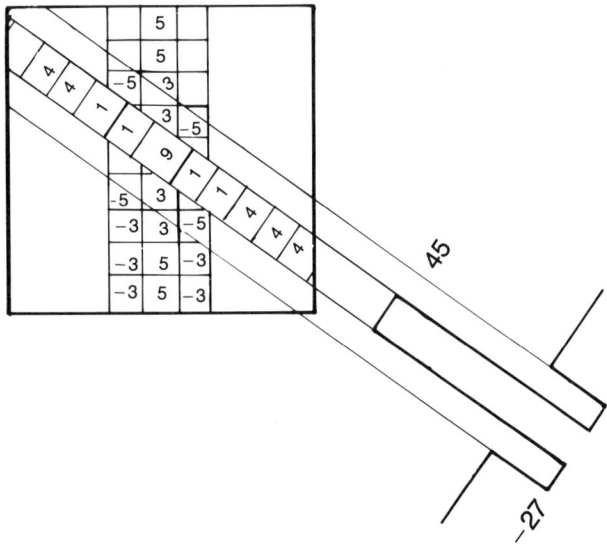

FIGURE 9-8 The second filtered projection profile is added onto the first profile in the image plane. Partial cancellation of streaks occurs with the summation of positive and negative values.

the first projection profile in the image plane. Notice that at the intersection of the projection lines with positive ray-sums, the pixel value became more positive when the counts were added together. In the two adjacent pixels where positive and negative values were combined, however, partial cancellation of the streaks occurred. Likewise, when the positive and negative ray-sums from the third projection profiles were added onto the image plane (Fig. 9-9), the point source image became more positive and there were more partial cancellations of the surrounding streaks. By acquiring more projection images at a number of angles around the point source, modifying the projection profiles with the same mathematical scheme, and then backprojecting the fudged projection profiles into the image plane, the negative side lobes cancelled more of the positive streaks. At the end, he obtained a reconstructed image of the point source with most of the streaks eliminated. This data fudging scheme (Fig. 9-6) is known as a convolution of the projection profile with a spatial filter, and the image reconstruction scheme is called the filtered backprojection method.

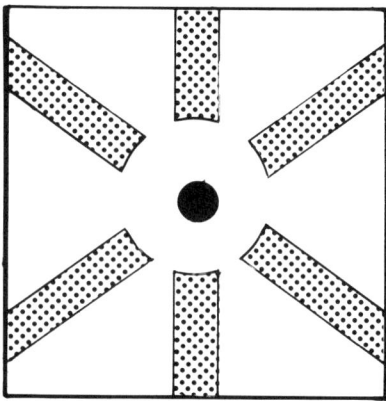

FIGURE 9-9 An isolated image of the point source is reconstructed after backprojecting the three filtered profiles in the image plane. The streak artifacts will be reduced further if more views of the point source were taken.

In the above example, mathematical accuracy was sacrificed in order to explain in an understandable fashion the concepts of filtered backprojection applied in the reconstruction of tomographic images. Of course, the appearance of the final image strongly depends on what the final projection profiles look like after modification of the original data with the "fudge" filters. Mathematical rigors are sacrificed again for a "look-see-do" approach to illustrate the strategy in selecting the optimal filter for reconstruction of tomographic images.

What Is That Window Doing on the Ramp?

According to high-power mathematics, the ideal reconstruction filter is the ramp filter if you can get multimillion counts in each projection profile. The ramp filter, when represented in the frequency domain, is a straight line as shown in Figure 9-10 that starts from zero and goes up linearly with the spatial frequency. The ramp filter, when transformed back to the spatial domain, look somewhat like the one shown in Figure 9-6 with two side lobes. For a review on the frequency description of an image, please refer to the discussion on Fourier analysis in Chapter 6.

SPECT

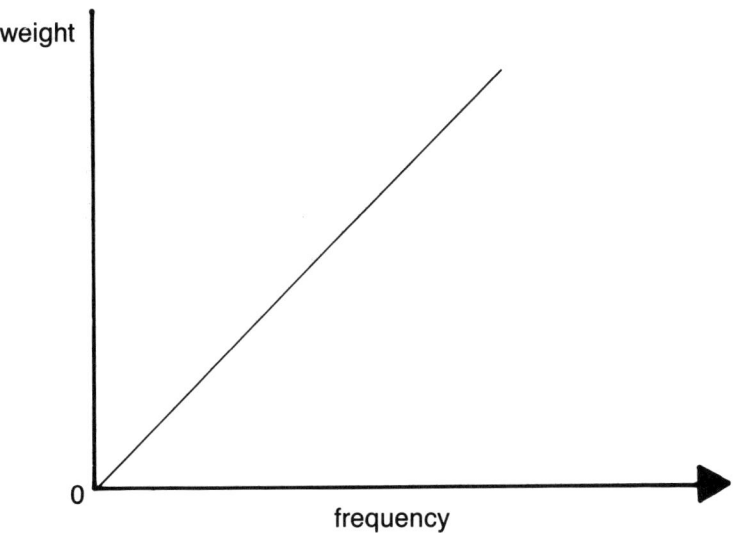

FIGURE 9-10 The ramp filter when plotted in the frequency domain is a straight line that starts from zero and increases linearly with frequency.

The ramp filter puts a low emphasis on the low-frequency components of the projection profile as compensation for redundant sampling of low-frequency data. On the other hand, the ramp filter heavily weighs the high frequency components to produce high resolution in the reconstructed image. If we have ideal projection data, we could reshape the projection profile with a ramp filter up to the Nyquist cut-off frequency (for now, the Nyquist cut-off frequency or the Nyquist frequency is defined as the maximum frequency resolvable by the camera computer system.) When we impose a range of frequencies to be included in the reconstruction, we are said to be modifying the ramp filter with a window function. The purpose of the window is to limit the reconstruction to data within a range of frequencies, analogous to the use of the energy window in the pulse-height analyzer of the gamma camera. Figure 9-11 shows a rectangular window that when superimposed on the ramp filter simply truncates the filter at the cut-off frequency. A rectangular window does not change the shape of the ramp; it merely sets a limit on the highest frequency to be included in the reconstruction.

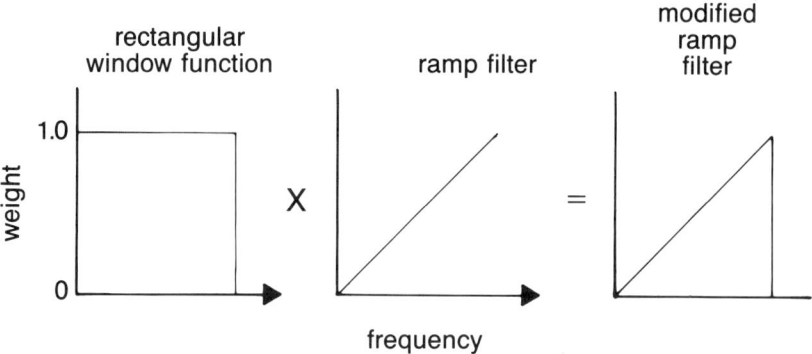

FIGURE 9-11 The rectangular window does not alter the characteristics of the ramp filter. It simply truncates the ramp filter at an upper frequency.

Figure 9-12 shows a transverse image of the liver reconstructed with a ramp filter that stops at the Nyquist frequency. The image is sharp but the edges are jagged, and there is noise scattered throughout the image much like some salt and pepper sprinkled in a bowl of soup. Such an image appearance is typical of using a ramp

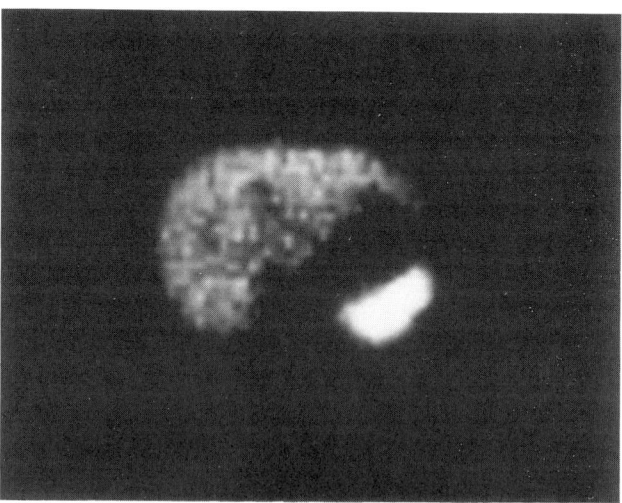

FIGURE 9-12 Images reconstructed with a ramp filter are unsatisfactory with much high frequency noise.

filter on clinical data with limited counts, especially in the high-frequency region. If the count statistics are low, the fraction of noise is high. Because the ramp filter preferentially amplifies high frequencies, the noise imbedded there is also greatly amplified. As a result, we end up with a high resolution image mingled with an exaggerated amount of noise. A different rectangular window can be used to truncate the ramp filter below the Nyquist frequency to reduce the amount of noise included in the reconstruction, but in so doing we may produce ring artifacts, i.e., fuzzy edges.

However, we can reduce noise without introducing artifacts by modifying the ramp filter with a window function that keeps the ramp filter intact in the low-frequency region, but gradually bends and flattens the ramp to zero at the cut-off frequency. The number of window functions devised for this purpose is considerable. One of the window functions commonly used in nuclear medicine is the Butterworth window (Fig. 9-13). In the low-frequency region, the coefficients on the Butterworth window is equal to 1.0. At about half way up to the Nyquist frequency, the curve takes on a fractional value and descends rapidly before gradually rolling to zero at the Nyquist frequency. When the ramp filter is modified by the coefficient of the Butterworth window at the corresponding frequency, the ramp remains unchanged in the low-frequency region because any num-

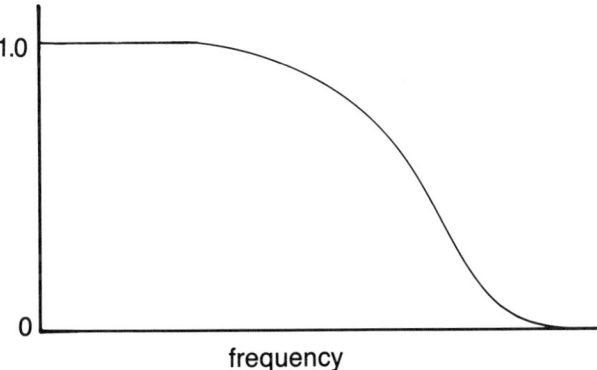

FIGURE 9-13 The Butterworth window starts with a weighting of 1.0 and rolls off from the cut-off frequency to zero at the Nyquist frequency. The steepness of decline is governed by the order of the Butterworth window.

ber multiplied by one is still the same number. Beginning at about one-half of the Nyquist frequency, the ramp is bent downward as a result of multiplication by a fraction. As the ramp continues onto the higher frequencies, the numerical value of the ramp is multiplied by a smaller and smaller fraction and eventually becomes zero at the Nyquist frequency. The last curve shown in Figure 9-14 is the composite filter after modifying the ramp filter with the Butterworth window. The composite filter is commonly known as the Butterworth filter, but "purists" will call it the Butterworth modified ramp filter. Figure 9-15 shows a transverse image of the liver reconstructed with the above Butterworth filter. Much of the "salt and pepper" noise was eliminated, but the spatial resolution was also reduced as evidenced by the smoother reconstructed image.

Figure 9-16 shows another Butterworth window with a cut-off frequency at one fourth of the Nyquist frequency. When this window is applied to the ramp filter, the resulting composite filter retains only the lowest frequencies for image reconstruction. Very little noise is evident in Figure 9-17, but oversmoothing also made the reconstructed image nearly useless. However, as shown in Figure 9-18, the same filter is well suited for reconstructing images in brain studies with ^{123}I-labeled amphetamine where the count statistics are much lower than those of liver studies.

In summary, the optimal reconstruction filter is a function of the count statistics; the higher the count statistics, then more high

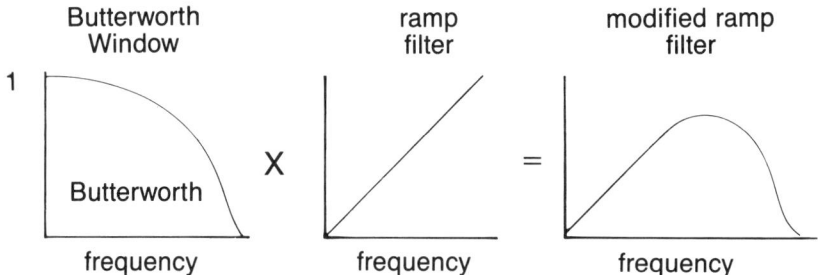

FIGURE 9-14 The ramp filter is modified by the Butterworth window with a cut-off frequency at 50% of the Nyquist frequency and an order of 5. The resulting ramp filter is unchanged in the low-frequency region, but the high frequencies are attenuated and reduced to zero at the Nyquist frequency.

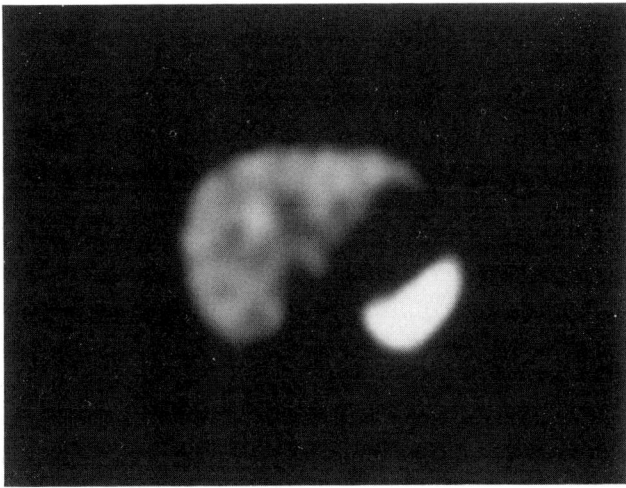

FIGURE 9-15 An image reconstructed with the Butterworth filter in Figure 9-14. Compared with images reconstructed with a ramp filter, the high-frequency noise was removed at the expense of reduced resolution.

frequencies can be included in the reconstruction. With a given filter, we can start the reconstruction with a high cut-off frequency. If the reconstructed image appears too fuzzy and grainy, drop the cut-off frequency to produce a smoother image. If oversmoothing occurred as a result of eliminating too many high frequencies, raise the cut-

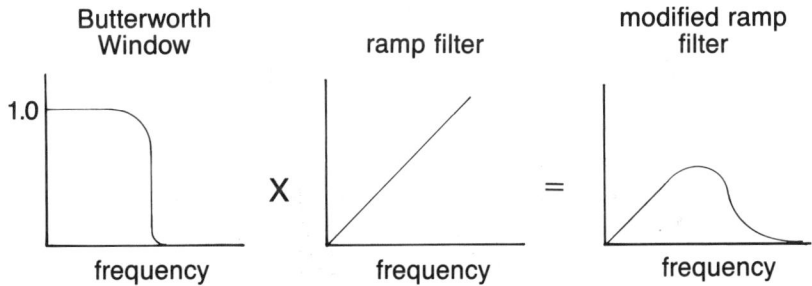

FIGURE 9-16 The ramp filter modified by a Butterworth window with a cut-off frequency at 25% of the Nyquist frequency and order 10. The resulting filter practically eliminated all the high frequency components in the projection images.

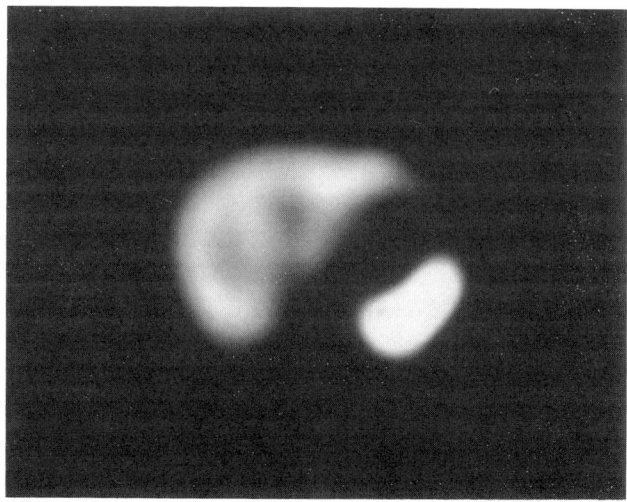

FIGURE 9-17 The Butterworth filter in Figure 9-16 produces an oversmoothed transfer image and is not useful clinically.

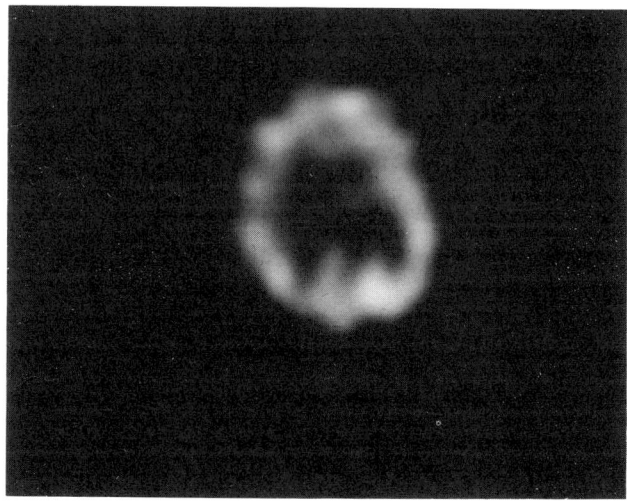

FIGURE 9-18 Due to an abundance of noise from poor count statistics, the Butterworth filter in Figure 9-16 produced a satisfactory image of ^{123}I-labeled iodoamphetamine in the brain.

off frequency and try again. The filter that we finally select is often the result of a subjective compromise between the amount of tolerable noise and the desirable resolution in the final image.

PHYSICAL FACTORS AFFECTING THE QUALITY OF SPECT IMAGES

In order to produce high quality SPECT images, we need to pay careful consideration to a number of factors during acquisition and processing of the projection images. During acquisition we need to ensure the accuracy of the gantry positioning and to optimize the angular and linear sampling frequencies for the type of clinical studies. In addition, we need to use the computer to process the data and the initial reconstructed images. Additional processings parameters include corrections for:

1. attenuation of the photons within the patient
2. inclusion of scattered photons in the projection images
3. variation of collimator resolution with depth
4. poor counting statistics
5. operational characteristics of the camera-computer system.

Linear Sampling Criteria

At each angular position of the gamma camera, the projection image is usually digitized by the computer to a 64 x 64 or 128 x 128 matrix. In SPECT, the exotic term *linear sampling* is used to describe the number of pixels in a row across the matrix. If the projection images are collected in a 64 x 64 matrix, there are 64 linear samples. Thus, the linear sample is the same as the linear dimension of the image matrix. Because each pixel is treated like a miniature radiation detector that measures the radioactivity lying along a line perpendicular to the pixel, the number of counts recorded in each pixel is called the ray-sum of the linear sample. A plot of the number of counts in each pixel along the row is called a projection profile. If we acquire an image in a 64 x 64 matrix, for instance, we obtain 64 projection profiles, each containing 64 linear samples or ray-sums. The maximum resolution obtainable in the reconstructed image can be inferred from the linear dimension of the matrix using the Nyquist sampling theorem which states that the maximum spatial frequency that we can observe is only half of the sampling frequency that we use to acquire the image. Suppose we take two measurements in each centimeter, the Nyquist sampling theorem says that the smallest lesion we can observe is one centimeter. Lesions smaller than one centimeter may not only be unresolvable due to inadequate sampling, but they may also introduce artifacts known as *aliases*.

In aliasing (Fig. 9-19), a wave of 9 cycles per centimeter appears as a different wave having 1 cycle per centimeter due to a low sampling frequency or to a lengthy sampling interval. For another example of aliasing, consider the rotation of a propeller on an airplane. We all know that the propeller blades turn in one direction only. However, as we watch the propeller start to turn, we see the blades turn faster and faster from rest. When it reaches a certain speed, it seems to turn in the opposite direction momentarily before our vision of the blades becomes completely blurred. This optical illusion is an example of aliasing. The propeller blades seem to rotate in the opposite direction because the sampling frequency of our eyes could not keep up with the rotational frequency of the propeller.

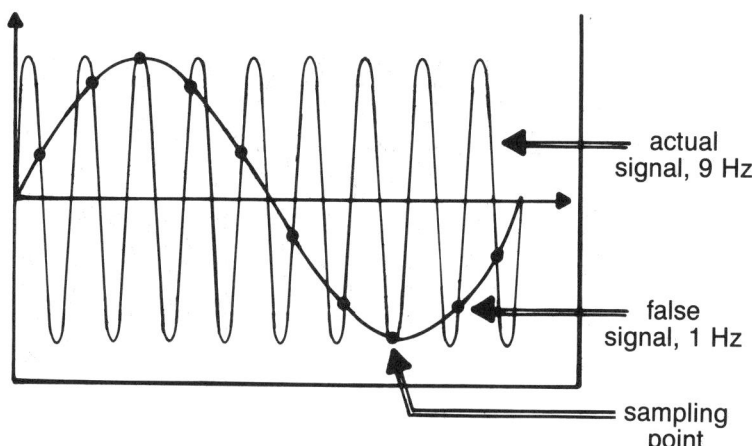

FIGURE 9-19 A 9-Hz input signal is mistakenly received as 1 Hz due to undersampling. False signals due to undersampling are called aliases.

If we treat a row of pixels in an image matrix as a row of sampling probes, the sampling frequency, **f**, is equal to the **n** number of pixels in the row divided by the diameter, **D**, of the field of view, (i.e., **f = n/D**). The highest observable spatial frequency, according to the Nyquist sampling theorem, is no greater than 0.5 **n / D**. As an example, suppose we use a camera with a 40-cm field of view to acquire an image onto a 64 x 64 matrix. The sampling frequency is f = 64/40 cm, or 1.6 cycles per centimeter; the space interval between samples is 0.625 cm. The Nyquist theorem says that we can only see at the most a spatial frequency of 0.8 cycles per centimeter, or a sample spacing of 1.25 cm. The higher frequencies present in the sample will not be seen or may appear as aliasing artifacts.

The Nyquist theorem tells us what image resolution to expect for a given sampling frequency under ideal conditions. We must not forget, however, that the spatial resolution of the gamma camera ultimately determines the maximum observable spatial frequency in the image. As a result the matrix size should be consistent with the spatial resolution of the gamma camera. Current state-of-the-art imaging with a 256 x 256 array is well within the spatial resolution of any modern gamma camera. However, a long imaging time is required in order to acquire a sufficient number of counts to keep statistical noise to an acceptable level. Also, image reconstruction time is greatly prolonged for the computer to process such large matrices. As a compromise to keep the statistical noise, acquisition time and computation time to a reasonable level, clinical tomographic images are usually acquired in 64 x 64 or 128 x 128 modes.

Angular Sampling Criteria

Image reconstruction theories assume that there are an infinite number of projections for reconstruction. In practice, only a finite number of projections are acquired. The number of angular samples taken is a compromise between the count density needed in each projection to keep image noise at an acceptable level and patient motion.

A number of empirical formulas have appeared in the literature to calculate the necessary number of angular views based on the size of the acquisition matrix and the diameter of the cross section to be imaged. Clinical images showed, however, that the angular sampling frequency can be smaller than those suggested by the empirical formulas and still produces an image of acceptable quality. Most commercial SPECT systems give the operator the option to acquire projection images from 2- to 10° increments over 360°. Since the imaging time is limited to about 30 minutes in order to reduce the patient motion, the acquisition time per view has to be reduced when the number of angular samples is increased. Thus, the time per view is 10 seconds when we acquire 180 images in 30 minutes, and increases to 50 seconds if we acquire only 36 views. Images reconstructed from phantom and patient studies acquired at 2° increments tend to be fuzzy due to a limited number of counts in each projection. With angular increments greater than 10°, annoying streak artifacts were seen in the reconstructed images. Angular samplings at 6° increments appeared to give the best compromise between statistical noise and streak artifacts.

Theoretically, we only need to acquire projection images over 180°. However, for most clinical studies, projections are acquired in stepwise rotation over 360°. One notable exception to 360° acquisition is thallium studies of the heart where errors due to scattering and internal absorption of the photons and nonuniform spatial resolution of the detector will off-set the advantage gained from complete angular sampling.

Photon Attenuation Correction

One of the fundamental assumptions of all SPECT reconstruction algorithms is that the ray-sum is directly proportional to the radioactivity along the ray. However, as the photons travel from their origin toward the camera, some are scattered away from the camera and some are absorbed by the intervening body tissues. Photons emitted from sites deep inside the body have a longer path of travel and are attenuated more than those near the body surface. As a result, the ray-sum is not linearly proportional to the quantity of radionuclide along the ray. If image reconstruction was done without correction for attenuation, a *hot rim* artifact is observed on the boundary of an organ, e.g., the anterior, posterior, and right lateral edges of the liver.

A number of methods have been developed to correct for photon attenuation. One approach incorporates a photon attenuation correction factor directly in the reconstruction algorithm. Due to its computational complexity, the development of this method has not received much momentum. A second approach corrects the projection data for attenuation prior to reconstruction. The simplest method in this category is to acquire data through 360° and use the geometric mean of the opposing projections for reconstruction. The geometric mean is calculated by taking the square root of the product of the two opposing ray-sums. This method of attenuation correction by averaging the conjugate ray-sums is easy to implement on the computer. However, the compensation is incomplete, and the reconstructed image require further modification in order to obtain sufficient degrees of spatial uniformity. Another method for tissue attenuation correction involves compensating each ray-sum by a factor proportional to the path-length of the photons from their origin to the body surface. This correction method requires knowledge of the body contour and assumes a constant attenuation coefficient within the body.

The third approach applies a correction factor to each pixel in the reconstructed image. This approach is a post-processing technique, i.e., after the transverse image is reconstructed. The correction factor for a given pixel in the reconstructed image is the average of the attenuation correction factors calculated for every ray passing through that image element. Assume that there are three rays passing through the point (x, y) in Figure 9-20. Because the pho-

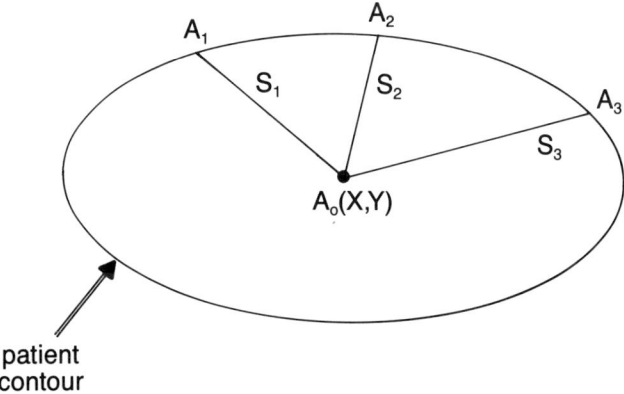

FIGURE 9-20 The post-processing method to correct for photon attenuation requires knowledge of the body contour.

tons originating from point (x, y) are attenuated as they travel to the detector, the measured activity at each projection is equal to the true activity Ao (x,y) at point (x, y) multiplied by an exponential attenuation factor:

$$A_1 = A_0(x,y)\exp(-\mu S_1)$$
$$A_2 = A_0(x,y)\exp(-\mu S_2)$$
$$A_3 = A_0(x,y)\exp(-\mu S_3)$$

where μ is the attenuation coefficient, S is the path-length of the photons and A_1, A_2 and A_3 are activities measured. We then assume that the calculated activity $A(x,y)$ in pixel (x,y) in the reconstructed image is equal to the average of the three measurements taken along rays S_1, S_2, and S_3:

$$A(x,y) = (A_1 + A_2 + A_3)/3$$

$$= A_0(x,y)\frac{\exp(-\mu S_1) + \exp(-\mu S_2) + \exp(-\mu S_3)}{3}$$

The true pixel value Ao (x,y) is obtained by re-arranging the above equation to give the following:

$$A_0(x,y) = \frac{3\,A(x,y)}{\exp(-\mu S_1) + \exp(-\mu S_2) + \exp(-\mu S_3)}$$

If the image was reconstructed using N number of projections, the correction factor should be multiplied by N instead of 3, and there should be N number of exponential terms in the denominator.

In summary, the activity $A(x,y)$ at pixel (x,y) should be corrected by an average attenuation correction factor to give

$$A_0(x,y) = C(x,y)\,A(x,y)$$

where

$$C(x,y) = \frac{N}{\sum_{i=1}^{n} \exp[-\mu S_i(x,y)]}$$

and $S_i(x,y)$ is the path-length of the photons from the point (x, y) to the edge of the body contour for the ith projection.

Keep in mind that the attenuation correction methods proposed thus far are approximate solutions to the problem. There are errors in determining the body contours and the assumption of a constant attenuation coefficient throughout the volume of reconstruction. Although we know that the attenuation coefficient varies for different types of tissues in the body, most attenuation correction methods suggest a constant value corresponding to the attenuation coefficient in water for the sake of simplicity. Satisfactory results were obtained for the head, abdomen and pelvis, but not for the thorax.

There are several proposed methods to measure the body contour. The simplest and the most commonly used method assumes that the body is an ellipse. The major and minor axes of the ellipse are defined by the distance between the image of two point sources placed on the anterior-posterior and the left-right lateral sides of the body section to be imaged. One of the techniques used to determine the body contour is by making a transverse section image of a ring of point sources placed around the body. Another technique utilizes projections of the Compton-scattered photons to form a transverse section image. Other methods use laser and ultrasound to scan around the patient to form the outline of the body. Presently, there is no concensus as to which is the best method for producing a body contour easily with minimum errors and in the shortest time.

Compton-Scattered Photons

Low-energy photons, such as those emitted from technetium-99m, lose only a small fraction of their energy as a result of small-angle scatter. Consequently, much of these small-angle scattered photons are able to pass through the pulse-height analyzer and get included in the projection images. The inclusion of scattered photons in the projection images not only degrades the image resolution, but also complicates the task of attenuation correction and other quantitative analyses on the reconstructed images.

Due to scattered photons that fall within the pulse-height analyzer window, the ray-sum is not a true representation of the total amount of activity along the ray. Because scattered photons increase the number of counts recorded in the ray-sum, the observed count rate of a point source does not drop off as rapidly with depth in the tissue as predicted by the exponential attenuation equation. For this reason, attenuation coefficient used in the attenuation correction methods is smaller than the value used for narrow monoenergetic beams. For example, the attenuation coefficient for the 140-keV photons from ^{99m}Tc in water is 0.15 cm^{-1} for a monoenergetic narrow beam geometry. To account for scattered photons in the data, the attenuation coefficient is empirically reduced to between 0.10 to 0.13 cm^{-1}.

The preferred method of scattered-photon rejection is to eliminate as much as possible those unwelcomed counts from getting recorded in the ray-sums. One method is to use an asymmetric energy window that is shifted toward the high energy end of the spectrum as in Figure 9-21. One of the two immediate consequences of using an off-peak window is a reduction of the count rate. As shown in Figure 9-21, the area bracketted by the asymmetric window under the photopeak is smaller than that by the usual symmetric win-

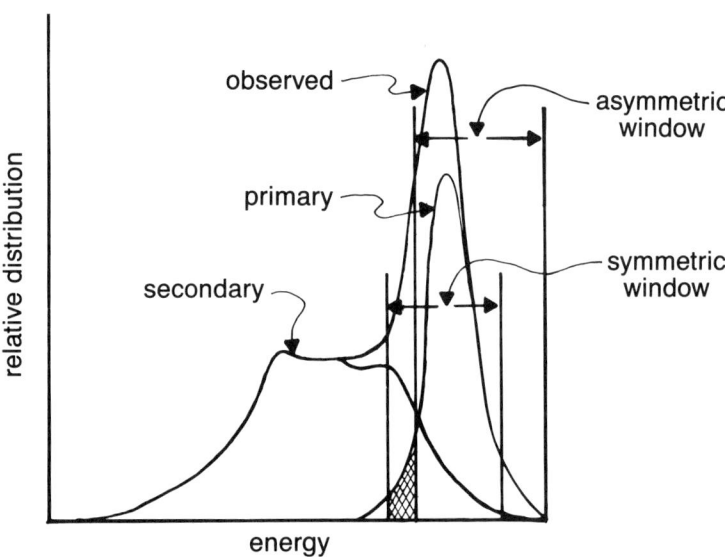

FIGURE 9-21 If the window of the pulse-height analyzer is set asymmetrically toward the high energy side, more scattered photons are eliminated at the expense of reduced count rate and possible distortion of the field uniformity.

dow. This means that many primary photons are sacrificed for a small reduction of the scattered photon contribution. In order to maintain the same statistical accuracy, a longer imaging time is needed to compensate for the reduced counting rate. Of course, whenever you lengthen imaging time, there is an increased risk of patient motion. The second and greater problem with using an asymmetric window is the risk of distorting the camera's field uniformity; creation of a nonuniform flood field on the camera is more deleterious to the image quality than the inclusion of scattered photons in the projection data.

Another approach to reducing the contribution of scattered photons might be to subtract from the projection image an image of the scattered-photon distribution using a window in the Compton region of the spectrum. However, studies have shown that Compton photons are not emitted isotropically. The energy and intensity of the Compton-scattered photons are different at different anatomical locations and at various projection angles around the body. Therefore, it is not a simple matter just to subtract the Compton image directly from the photopeak image and arrive at a so-called "scatter-free" image.

There are a number of other techniques in the literature to correct for scattered photons in the gamma camera images. However, no Compton correction technique is satisfactory so long as we continue to use the NaI detector that exhibits an energy resolution of 10%-15%. Solid-state detectors have energy resolution an order of magnitude greater than that of the NaI. Unfortunately, problems with cryogenic cooling and the unavailability of a large crystal preclude their use clinically.

Non-Circular Detector Motion

Another fundamental assumption of the reconstruction algorithm is that the width of each ray remains constant at all distances from the detector. This assumption is flagrantly violated when using the gamma camera as the detector. Each projected ray on a gamma camera is defined by the field of view of channels in the collimator. Figure 9-22 shows that the field of view of a collimator channel diverges as the distance from the face of the collimator increases.

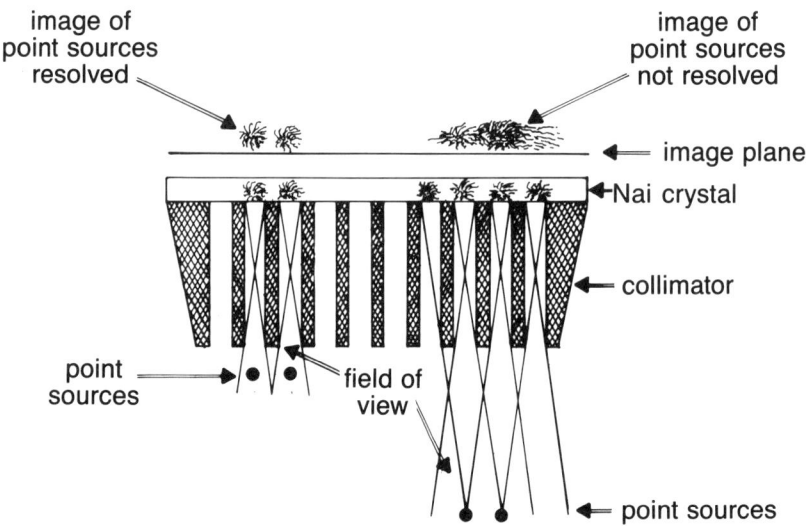

FIGURE 9-22 Two point sources become indistinguishable when they are moved to a distance away from the surface of collimator.

Therefore, the structures deep inside the body are not as well resolved as those near the body surface. If the gamma camera follows a circular orbit around the patient as shown in Figure 9-23, the patient's position is first adjusted so that the axis of rotation coincide with the midline of the body. The radius of rotation, (i.e., the distance of the gamma camera from the axis of rotation) is then adjusted to clear the patient's shoulders or hips. Figure 9-23 shows that the face of the collimator is located much farther away from the patient in the anterior and posterior positions than in the left-right positions. Therefore, the resolution of the gamma camera images are worse in the anterior-posterior positions than in the lateral orientations. In fact, the image resolution continuously changes as a function of the angular position of the gamma camera.

Every SPECT system provides the user with options, such as the body contour following method shown in Figure 9-24 or an elliptical orbit, to continuously adjust the detector's radius of rotation to minimize patient-to-detector distance. Regardless of the method used, all must conform to the assumptions used in the reconstruction algorithm. First, the axis of rotation must remain fixed at one position inside the body. Second, the face of the collimator

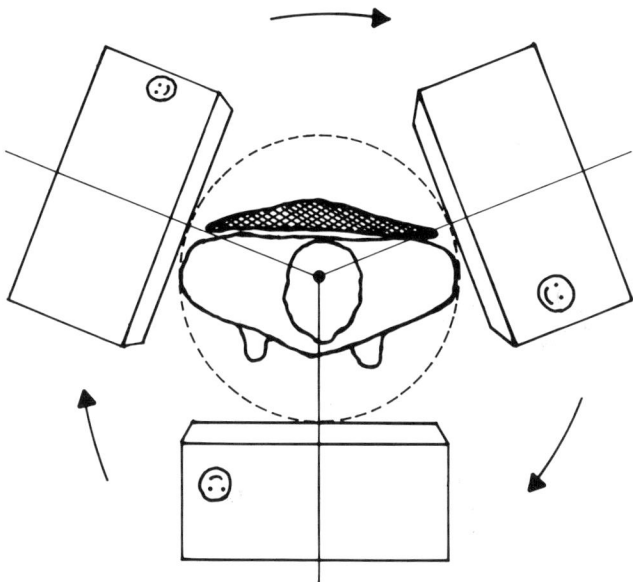

FIGURE 9-23 In a circular orbit, the gamma camera is farther away from the patient in the anterior and posterior positions than in the lateral positions.

must be perpendicular to the radius of rotation at all angular positions. Finally, each angular increment of the detector must be equal. Therefore, whenever one of the non-circular camera motions is used during acquisiton, the resulting projection image must be corrected to conform with the above assumptions prior to reconstruction.

Clinical trials with acquiring projection images using non-circular detector motion showed rather disappointing results. The conclusions were that too much time was spent setting up the camera and preparing the patient for imaging, total imaging time also was increased because the detector and table need to adjusting to different positions at each projection angle, and that while extra time was required for data processing, the resulting reconstructed images did not show any real improvement over the usual circular detector motion. The reason for the disappointing results might be that the data acquired from a non-circular orbit must be corrected to conform with assumptions used in the reconstruction algorithm. Evidently, the slight gain in image resolution from moving the collimator close

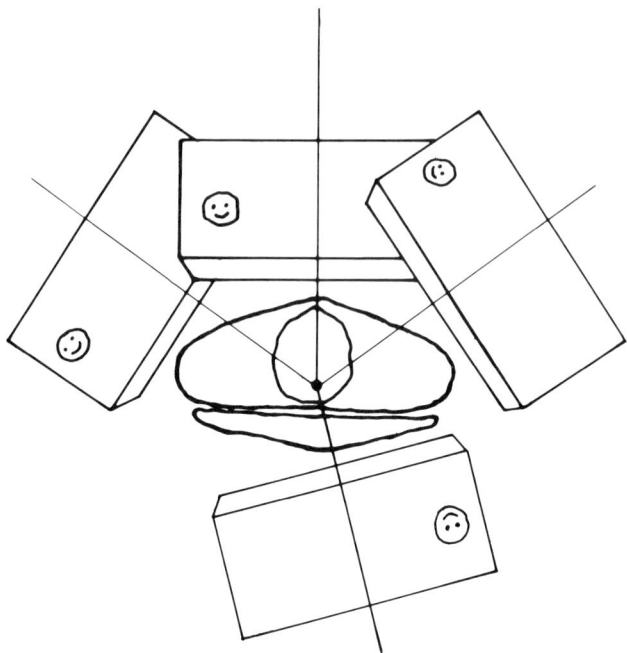

FIGURE 9-24 The non-circular detector motion attempts to bring the gamma camera as close to the patient as possible at each projection angle.

close to the patient was off-set by errors resulting from the translations, interpolations, and averaging of the projection data before reconstruction.

Image Noise

Several empirical equations have been proposed to quantify noise in the reconstructed images. Instead of going into a detailed discussion on empirical equations, those factors contributing to image noise are presented. After all, these equations only attempt to link the different physical factors together with a weighting factor to arrive at a numerical index of the image noise.

The major source of image noise is the limited number of counts in a reconstructed image. If we say that conventional planar images are *photon-limited*, then SPECT images are *photon-starved*. As a comparison, a planar image generally contains 500,000 counts, while a SPECT image contains only about 200,000 counts. Based on the ratio of counts alone, SPECT images already have 60% greater noise than planar images.

$$(\sqrt{500{,}000/200{,}000} = 1.6\%).$$

Patients undergoing SPECT scans are routinely given a dose 30%-50% higher than that for planar imaging in order to increase the photon flux without prolonging the imaging time. There are SPECT systems, such as the one shown in Figure 9-25, that use

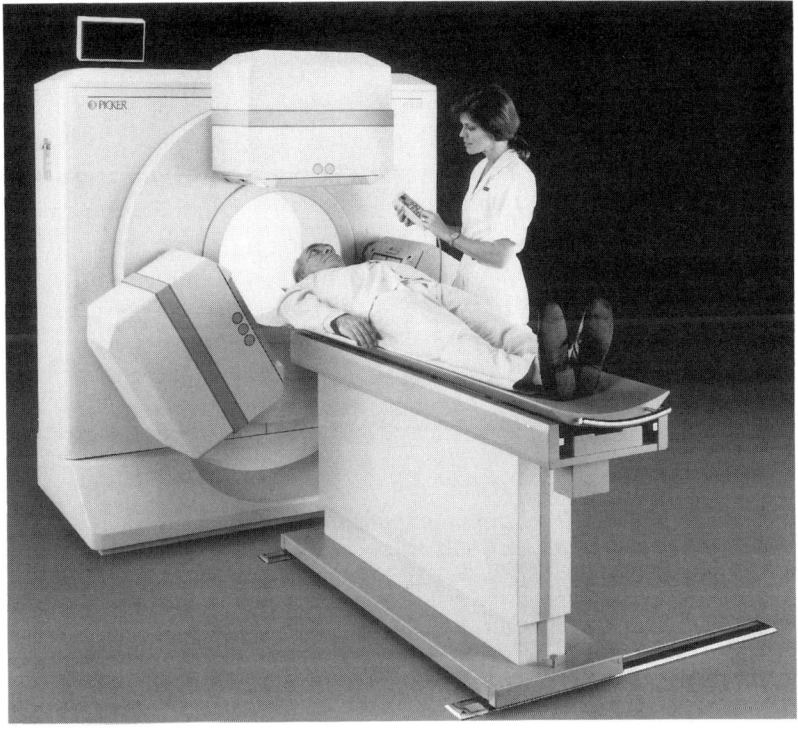

FIGURE 9-25 SPECT systems with three detectors will be able to collect more counts, hence higher image resolution, in the same imaging time as a single detector system. (Reprinted courtesy of Picker Inc.).

three gamma camera detectors and other systems that use two detectors to collect counts simultaneously to increase the counting statistics within the same data collection time. The multi-detector approach is useful on scans with low counting rates, but it also demands greater quality control. Perhaps one of the long-term solutions to photon famine is the development of detectors with higher detection efficiency.

Increasing the number of pixels in the acquisition matrix will increase resolution, but statistical noise in each pixel will be increased concomitantly if the total number of counts acquired per projection remains constant. Therefore, we must not forget the simple rule that whenever the matrix dimension is doubled, the number of counts acquired into the matrix must be quadrupled in order to keep pixel noise unchanged.

Random noise is an important, but not the only, source of noise in a reconstructed image. There is propagation of noise resulting from the reconstruction algorithm, window function, the size and shape of the region to be reconstructed, the pixel size, as well as linear and angular sampling errors. The noise level is different from pixel to pixel and is greater in the interior portion of the reconstructed image than in the peripheries, a result due to the noise amplification characteristics of the image reconstruction algorithm.

QUALITY ASSURANCE OF THE SPECT SYSTEM

Many of physical factors affecting the quality of SPECT images are similar to those affecting planar gamma camera images. This fact should not be surprising since the tomographic images are derived mathematically from the planar images. However, a much more rigorous control of camera-computer performance is required for SPECT imaging than for conventional planar imaging. It has been shown theoretically and verified experimentally that image reconstruction is a noise amplification process. During reconstruction, small errors in the projection images can be amplified in to severe artifacts in reconstructed images. The problem with error amplification is particularly severe for high frequency components and noise close to the axis of rotation.

SPECT

Because the image reconstruction process amplifies and propagates noise and errors imbedded in the projection images, the gamma camera system for SPECT imaging requires more stringent quality assurance than cameras for planar imaging. Also, the quality assurance procedures for planar imaging were designed for a single measurement with the detector stationary at one fixed orientation. While the measurement provides a good indication of tomographic image quality, the results may not apply when the detector is rotated to other orientations during image acquisition. For example, it was discovered in the early days of SPECT that the energy response of the photomultiplier tubes actually varied as a function of its orientation relative to the earth's magnetic field. Although the subtle angular variation of the energy response of the photomultiplier tubes did not affect the quality of planar images, noticeable ring artifacts were produced on the SPECT images.

In spite of the absence of any well-accepted quality assurance protocols and equipment performance standards for SPECT systems, several factors have been recognized as important for producing high-quality SPECT images: (1) camera field uniformity, (2) center of rotation, (3) pixel size, and (4) alignment of the pixel axes.

Camera Field Uniformity

Studies have shown that a 1% nonuniformity in the planar images can be amplified to as much as 20% nonuniformity near the axis of rotation in the recontructed image. Hence, each planar projection image must be corrected for sensitivity variation across the field of view of the gamma camera prior to reconstruction of the transaxial images. The correction is done by creating a matrix of multiplication factors to modify the number of counts in the corresponding pixels in the projection images. This matrix of correction factors is derived from the image of a uniform flood source which has less than 1% variation in its activity distribution.

The fillable flood phantom for uniformity tests for planar imaging gamma camera is unsatisfactory. There are no adequate ways to ensure that the inserted ^{99m}Tc activity is uniformly mixed to within 1% with the water inside. Because the surfaces of the phantom are bowed under the weight of the water, we have to press the surfaces with, for example, a pair of hard boards to make them flat.

In so doing, water is ocassionally squirted out from the phantom, thereby creating a radiation contamination problem: there is no guarantee that the phantom surfaces become flat to within 1% either.

Cobalt-57 flood sources are commercially available with a guaranteed activity uniformity to within 1%. The ^{57}Co flood sources are obviously more convenient to use because they eliminate the laborious filling procedure and the associated radiation safety problems. However, the maximum activity in a typical ^{57}Co flood source is about 5 mCi. Consequently, the acquisition time when using a ^{57}Co phantom is considerably longer than when using 7-10 mCi of ^{99m}Tc in a fillable phantom. Also, the imaging time continually increases due to radioactive decay of the ^{57}Co, and the costly phantom needs to be replaced at least every 2 years in order to keep the image acquisition time to within an acceptable length.

Since radioactive decay is a stochastic process, the need to achieve a statistical uncertainty of less than 1% in the flood image will require at least 10,000 counts to be acquired into each pixel in the flood image. For a 64 x 64 matrix circumscribing the camera field of view, there are 3217 pixels in the flood image, i.e., the number of pixels N in a circle is

$$N = \pi(d/2)^2$$
$$N = \pi(64/2)^2$$
$$= 3217$$

When we multiply the 3217 pixels by 10,000 counts per pixel, we get approximately 30 million as the number of counts needed for the flood correction matrix. For a 128 x 128 matrix, there are four times as many pixels in the image and, hence, 120 million counts will be needed in order to keep the statistical noise to within 1%. The acquisition time for such a large number of counts usually takes up to several hours when using a ^{59}Co flood phantom.

It must be emphasized that a given correction matrix is applicable only to data acquired under the same conditions as the flood image. For example, patient images must be acquired with the same collimator attached to the detector in the same orientation, using the same matrix size and zoom factor. Ideally a new uniformity correction matrix should be created for each isotope energy. Due to the long time involved with acquiring the flood images, the uniforty correction matrix created with ^{59}Co is assumed to be applicable at other energy windows. For the current generation of gamma cameras with built-in energy and linearity correction circuits, the energy response of the camera across its field of view does not seem to vary tremendously with different energy windows. At the time of equipment acceptance testing, camera uniformity could be tested at different energies, but it need not be done routinely. During acceptance testing, flood images should be taken at several gantry angles to test for collimator shift and the influence of the gravitation and external electromagnetic fields on the detector response.

Center of Rotation

Image reconstruction theory assumes that when a ray is projected from the center of the detector at each angle, these rays intersect at a common point known as the center of rotation (Fig. 9-26). The axis of rotation is an imaginary line drawn through the COR about which the detector rotates. The pixel in the image matrix corresponding to this COR, therefore, needs to be identified in order for the software to perform the image reconstruction.

The center of rotation in the projection image matrix can be derived from two images of a point source, each taken 180° apart. As shown in Figure 9-26, the two opposing images of a point source are located at a equal distance from the COR. In other words, the center of rotation is located at the pixel halfway between the two pixels occupied by the point source image in the opposing views. For example, if the image of the point source is located at pixel number 17 in projection A, and is located at pixel 47 in the opposing projection C, then the COR is located at pixel 32, the average of the two pixel numbers. Usually 30 pairs of such images are acquired to calculate 30 values of the center of rotation. The average of these 30 values is used as the COR for subsequent image reconstructions.

Pixel Size

Accurate calibration of the pixel size is necessary for photon attenuation correction and for measurement of organ or lesion volume. The dimensions of a pixel can be easily measured by taking an image of two point sources located at a known distance apart. For a

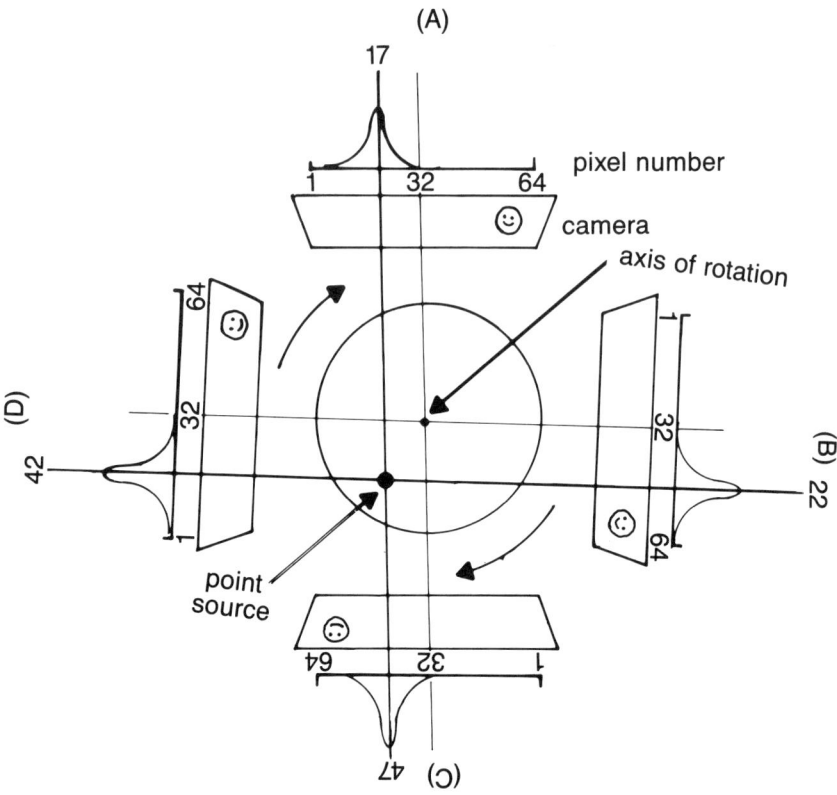

FIGURE 9-26 The COR is calculated by taking the average of the pixel numbers under the peak of the activity profile of a point source in the opposing views.

40-cm useful field of view, we can place two point sources on the collimator at 25 cm apart. The common ^{57}Co disk markers make ideal point sources for this purpose, as they can be easily placed at a desired location. Alternatively, we can substitute the ^{57}Co marker sources with two glass capillary tubes, each containing a small quantity of ^{99m}Tc in it. Of course, we must make sure that the ^{99m}Tc solution does not leak from the glass tubes and contaminate the collimator.

Once an image of the two point or line sources has been acquired, the pixel location of each source in the computer image is identified from the activity profile as shown in Figure 9-27. The pixel

SPECT

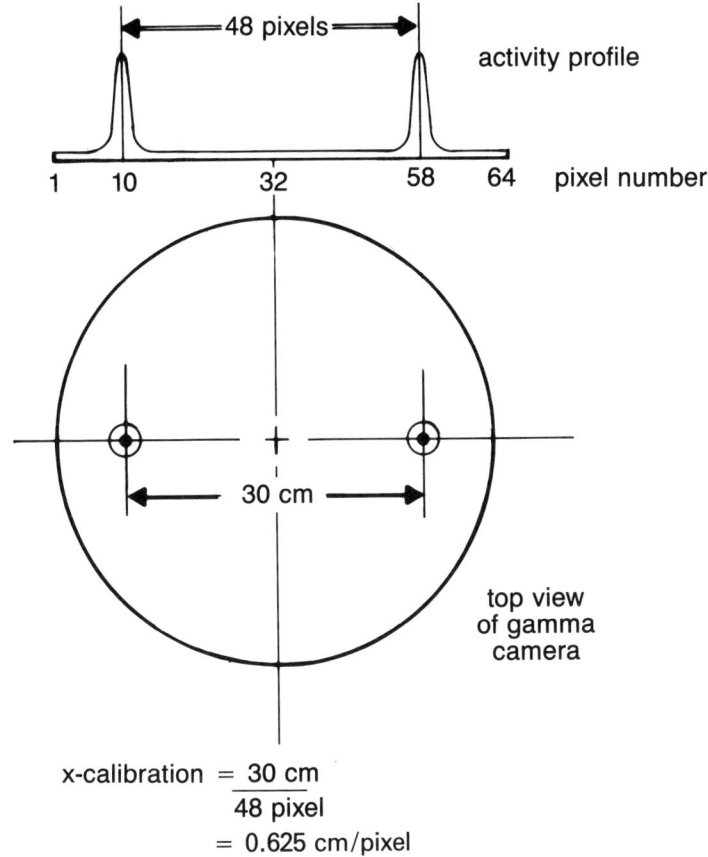

FIGURE 9-27 The dimensions of a pixel is determined by dividing the separation distance between two point sources by the number of pixels between the peaks in the projection profile.

dimension is calculated by dividing the separation distance between the two point sources by the number of pixels between the two peaks in the activity profile of the image in the illustration. If the image of the two point sources were acquired in a 64 x 64 array using a 40-cm useful field of view gamma camera, the linear dimension of a pixel is nominally equal to 6.25 mm; for a 128 x 128 image matrix, it is equal to 3.13 mm.

The pixel dimension must be calibrated in both the x and y axes of the camera's field of view. It is easy to make adjustments on the gain or amplification of the and positional signals so that the number of millimeters per pixel in the two perpendicular directions are equalized to within 2% of each other. For precise calculation of organ or lesion volume from tomographic images, the known pixel dimensions will need to be better than 0.5 mm.

Orthogonality and Centering

By adjusting the offset control of the x and y positional signals from the gamma camera, the axes of the image matrix can be calibrated to intersect at the exact midpoint (i.e., if the offset control of the camera's position signal is well adjusted, the center of the camera's field of view for a 128 x 128 image matrix, for example, should be located at pixel 64 on both the and axes). The axes centering procedure can also be easily done using five ^{57}Co point sources as shown in Figure 9-28. With most gamma cameras the location of each photomultiplier tube is marked by a dot on the protective cover of the crystal. By placing a source over the location of the central photomultiplier and two sources at equidistant from the central point source along each of the orthogonal axes passing through center, the image acquired into the computer will allow profiles to be drawn and analyzed regarding the symmetry, othogonality, and gain of the and axes.

CONCLUSION

In this chapter, a brief explanation of the computer methods involved in the acquisition, processing, and quality assurance of a SPECT system have been presented. One of the nice features of commercial SPECT systems is that they all try to shield complicated mathematical and computer details from the users. In so doing, technologists can concentrate on ways to optimize patient studies and not get bogged down in a neverending dialogue with a temperamental computer. Hopefully the materials discussed in this chapter will enable the reader to better understand the reasoning behind many manufacturers' software protocols.

SPECT

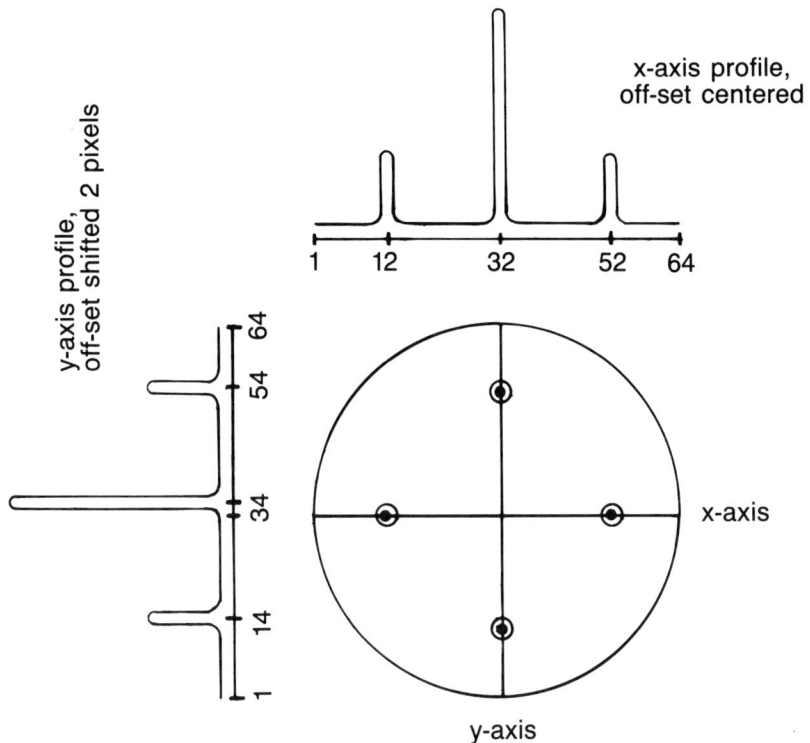

FIGURE 9-28 If the off-sets of the x and y axes were properly adjusted, a point source placed in the center of the crystal should produce a peak in the activity profile in the center pixel of the image matrix. By acquiring an image of five point sources (one at the center and two pairs at known distances apart along the x and y axes), the offsets and pixel dimensions can be measured simultaneously.

SUGGESTED READINGS

1. AAPM Report Number 22. Rotating scintillation camera SPECT acceptance testing and quality control. American Institute of Physics, Inc., 1987.

2. Array AP.Processing in medical imaging. *IEEE Computer.* 1983;16:17-30.

3. Bieszk JA, Hawman EG. Evaluation of SPECT angular sampling effects: continuous versus step-and-shoot acquisition. *J Nucl Med* 1987;28:1308-1314.

4. Brooks RA, DiChiro G. Principles of computer-assisted tomography (CAT) in radiographic and radioisotopic imaging. *Phys Med Biol* 1976;21:689-731.

5. Budinger TF. Physical attributes of single-photon tomography. *J Nucl Med* 1980;21:579-592.

6. Eisner RJ. Principles of instrumentation in SPECT. *J Nucl Med Technol* 1985;13:23-31.

7. Greer K, Jasczak R, Harris C, Coleman E. Quality control in SPECT. *J Nucl Med Technol* 1985;13:76-159.

8. King MA, Doherty PW, Rosenberry RJ, Cool SL. Array processors: an introduction to their architecture, software, and applications in nuclear medicine. *J Nucl Med* 1983;24:1027-1079.

9. Murase K, Itoh H, Mogami H, et al. A comparative study of attenuation correction algorithms in single-photon emission computed tomography (SPECT). *Eur J Nucl Med* 1987;13:55-62.

10. Rogers WL, Clinthorne BA, Harkness BA, Koral KF, Keyes JW. Field flood requirements for emission computed tomography with an anger camera. *J Nucl Med* 1982;23:162-168.

CHAPTER

10

AN ALL DIGITAL NUCLEAR MEDICINE DEPARTMENT

INTRODUCTION

Since the mid-1980s, the use of computers has been greatly expanded for radionuclide imaging. It is now common to find two or more computers in use in nuclear medicine departments. However, the proliferating use of computers also brought about problems with accessing images that were aquired and/or processed in different computers. In fact, it is frustrating to either scurry from one computer to another to search for a given patient's images, or be unable to display, much less process, a set of patient images because it was acquired on another computer with different hardware and software configurations.

Computer networking is an emerging technology which seeks to solve the problems of information exchange and equipment sharing between computers. Achieving this goal demands both proper physical linkage of different types of computers as well as sophisticated software that allows users to access the network, transmit, and receive data in an efficient and orderly fashion. In this chapter, the essential features of a computer network, particularly the picture archival and communication system (PACS), used to facilitate storage, retrieval, and display of the radionuclide images between computers, are discussed.

COMMUNICATION NETWORKS

One distinct characteristic of a computer network is that images are moved electronically from one computer to another for processing, interpretation by the physician, or for archiving and making hardcopy documentation. The electronic interconnection of the different hardware devices in the acquisition, processing, archiving, hardcopy documentation, and viewing stations is called the communication network, computer network, or just network for short. Each station in the computer network is called a network node.

There are two broad categories of computer networks: the wide area network (WAN) and the local area network (LAN). The computers in a WAN could use microwave and satellite to communicate with each other at hundreds and thousands of miles apart, while the LAN utilizes cables to physically link together computers located within a few thousand feet from each other, usually within a building. LANs are used for communicating digital images between the different nodes in a nuclear medicine department.

Network Transmission Medium

Network transmission medium is a fancy term used to describe the type of cables used for conveying digital information in a computer network. A simple connector is a parallel cable (Fig. 10-1A) which is a flat cable made up of several wires each carrying one bit of information. The multi-wire ribbon cable connecting the printer to the computer is one example of a parallel transmission medium. Unfortunately, a parallel cable, as it runs through the building, easily picks up electrical noises such as those coming from the elevators, fluorescent lights, power lines, and motors.

A more noise-tolerant medium is a pair of twisted wires, similar to those twisted wires in telephone cables. These twisted wires (Fig. 10-1B) also pick up noise, but because each wire in the twisted pair picks up noise nearly equally, the noise can be summed up and cancels each other at the end of transmission.

Another method is the use of a coaxial cable (Fig. 10-1C) with a center conductor completely shielded by a metallic mesh that blocks out undesired electrical noise. Coaxial cables, when compared to parallel cables, have the advantages of low noise and fewer number

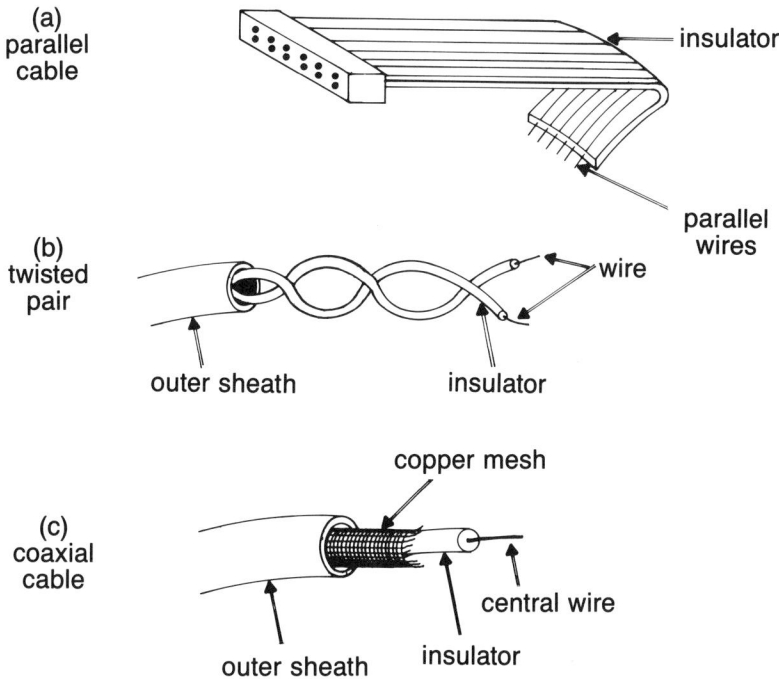

FIGURE 10-1 Parallel cables (A) are used for communication between components within a computer. They are not used in a LAN due to its susceptibility to electrical noise. The twisted pair of wires (B) and coaxial cables (C) are common network transmission mediums.

of connecting wires; the disadvantage is that they contain only one wire for the passage of electrical signals. As a result, data must be transmitted one bit after another in serial form. If we want to transmit multiple signals of different kinds, such as voice, text, and video information, through the coaxial cable simultaneously, we will need a complicated mechanism known as *multiplexing*, which will be discussed in the next section.

Fiber optics are immune to surrounding electrical noise and transmit data faster than electrical cable schemes. Unlike cables, which transmit information by variations of electrical voltage, fiber optics relay information by using variations of light intensity traveling through a fiber optic rod. Conceptually, data transmission via fiber optics (Fig. 10-2) is very simple. When light traveling in one medium encounters a second medium with a lower optical density (or refractive index), some of the incident light is bounced back to the original medium. If the light hits the boundary at a relatively shallow angle with respect to the direction of travel, a large fraction of the incident light is reflected back to the first medium. By making a glass fiber where the core has a greater optical density than the outer layer, light can be sent through a curved fiber at 100 megabits per second for miles with hardly any loss of intensity. In principle, a fiber optic cable can replace a wire simply by using a device that converts variations of electrical voltage into corresponding variations of light intensity. However, the cost of this speedy and yet low-noise network medium is still expensive at the present time. Hence, coaxial cables are widely used as the compromise between cost, noise, and speed.

Methods of Data Transmission

When using coaxial cables, twisted pairs of wires, or fiber optic cables to link together the nodes in a local area network, we can use either the *baseband* or the *broadband* methods for transporting data from one node to another. The baseband method uses a digital technique to send signals one at a time through the cable, while the broadband method uses an analog technique to send multiple signals through a single cable at the same time.

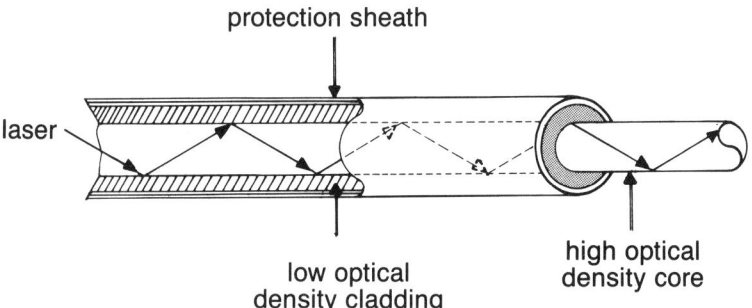

FIGURE 10-2 A fiber-optic cable consists of a bundle of glass fibers in the core and a surrounding cladding of higher optical density. A laser device encodes the information as pulses of light sends it through the cable as fast as 100 megabits per second.

The connecting cable in a baseband network serves as the communication channel for digital voltage pulses to propagate from one node to the other. Because there is only one communication channel available in a baseband network, only one message at a time is allowed on the network cable. Hence, the nodes have to wait their turn to transmit. However, the baseband method is simple. Because of its simplicity, the baseband is the preferred method of data transmission when system reliability is of prime consideration. Also, due to the lower cost, most LANs operate in the baseband.

The broadband transmission method uses a technique called multiplexing to divide a single communication cable into a number of channels for simultaneous transmission of analog signals at different frequencies. The range of frequencies allowed to travel in the network cable is called the *bandwidth*. In a broadband network, several different signals can transmit simultaneously using different portions of the bandwidth—not separate cables. Thus, the wider the bandwidth, the greater the variety and quantity of information can be sent through the network at any one time. This is the same technique used by the cable television industry to allow multiple television channels to share the same cable set. The subscribers can select from several different television channels, each broadcasting at the same time on its own designated frequency. Because of the complexity and cost of the network components required to convert signals back and forth between the digital and analog forms, broadband networks are generally employed in large buildings, or in a WAN so that users over a wide geographic area can access a variety of information quickly.

LOCAL AREA NETWORK TOPOLOGY

Because the baseband transmission method employed in most LANs has only a single channel, data communication through the network must be done using serial transmission protocols. When more than two computers are connected together in a network using a serial line, a method must be devised to determine which node in the network has the right to use the network at any given moment. A right-to-use protocol is needed because with a single serial line, only one computer can transmit at a given time. While one computer is using the network, all other computers in the network must wait for its turn. The computer inter-connection schemes that have been devised to accomodate the serial transmission protocols generally fall under three main categories or topologies: star, ring, or bus network as shown in Figure 10-3.

Star Network

In the star configuration, each computer is connected via cable to a central computer called the network server to direct communication traffic in the network. To communicate with any computer in the network, a signal must first be sent to the central computer asking for permission to transmit. If the network is busy, the caller is placed on hold, in queue, until the communication traffic is clear. When the line is free, the central computer then alerts the destination computer that a message is on the way and makes the switch which allows data transmission to begin. The concept of star network resembles the old-time private-branch-exchange (PBX) telephone system with a central switch board. In order to talk to a person on the telephone using the PBX system, the caller must contact the switch board operator, who first checks to see if the line is open, and then makes the switch connection. Star network has two shortcomings. First, the central computer is busy monitoring communication traffic and is not able to do anything else. Second, if the central switching computer fails, then the entire network fails. The advantages of a star network are its simplicity and inexpensiveness. The star network is thus attractive for the interconnection of computers in a small offfice or a nuclear medicine department with relatively few users.

Ring Network

Computers in a ring network are connected to each other to form a closed loop. A more sophisticated ring network include two loops with data moving in clockwise and counter-clockwise directions. Unlike the star network, all nodes in the ring network share the responsibility for maintaining the communication activities, instead of relying on one central computer as is the case of a star network. One of the advantages of a ring network is that the loop circumference

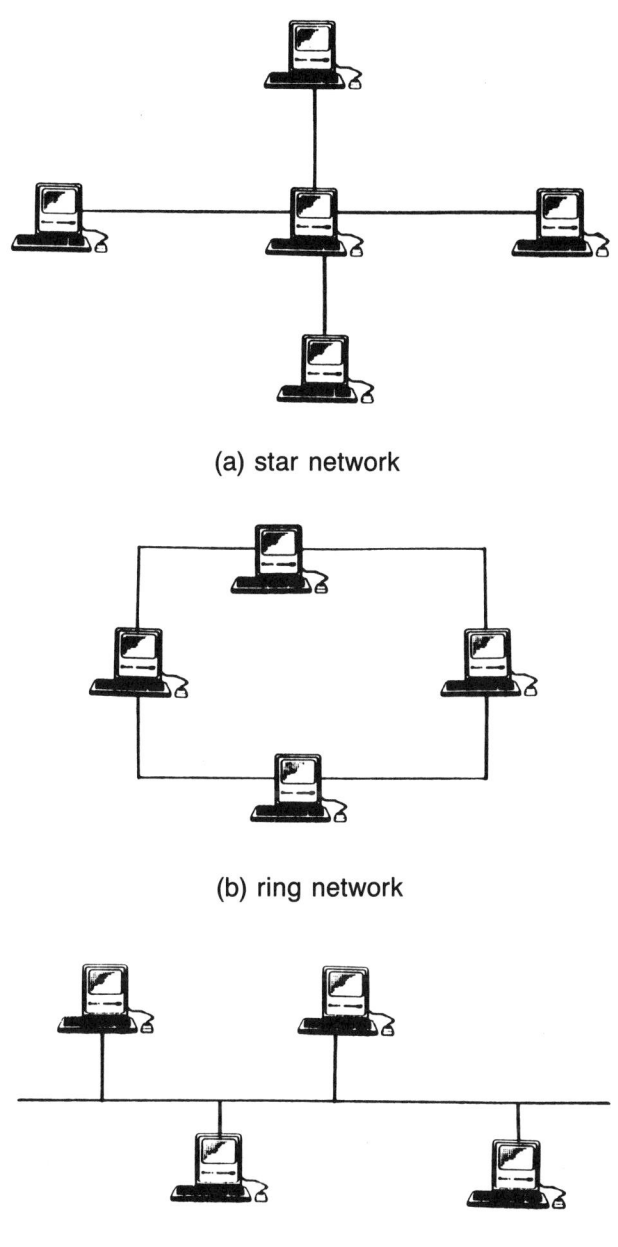

(a) star network

(b) ring network

(c) bus network

FIGURE 10-3 The three general methods for the linking of the computers in a LAN.

can be extended to several hundred thousand feet, thus enabling linkage of a number of computers over a large area. In case one node fails, however, the loop is broken and the network will shut down. When this happens, the malfunctioning equipment in the node can be bypassed to reactivate the network with the other functional nodes. The main disadvantage with the ring configuration is the difficulty with modifying the number of nodes and locations of the nodes in the ring. If a new node is to be added to the ring, new cables must be connected between the new node and its two adjacent nodes. It is also expensive to alter the node locations in an existing ring network because many cables need to be re-routed.

Another name for the ring network is the token-ring network because it uses the token passing method to gain control of the network for data transmission. The token passing method continuously circulates an empty token, which is a unique 8-bit pattern, around the network to each station. Any station can grab the empty token to gain access to the network, attach it with data, and let it continue on its route. Every station is given an identification address and when a loaded token passes by that destination address, the data is unloaded and acknowledged by the receiving station. The empty token is then sent onto the next station, etc. If the station has no message to send when the token arrives, it simply waives its chance and the token moves on to the next station. An empty token passes by each network station at regular time intervals, thus guaranteeing each station their own regular opportunities to use the network. Also, the high regularity of data traffic reduces the rate of error occurence.

Bus Network

Bus topology involves one long central data transmission cable called a network bus. A number of nodes are connected to this main distribution channel. Some sophisticated bus configurations incorporate two cables running from each node; one cable receives while the other cable transmits. Similar to the nodes in a ring network, each node in the bus network has its own data communication module. Unlike the ring or star networks, however, in the case that one or more nodes in the network fail, the network still stays active by serving the other functional nodes. Another advantage of the bus configuration is the ease with which new nodes can be added or existing nodes be removed without disturbing the data communication activities in the network. They are the two main reasons why most pilot PACS use the bus configuration for digital imaging network. Although the token passing method can be used, bus networks utilize the carrier sense multiple access method (CSMA) for data communication. With the CSMA method, a node wanting to use the network for data transmission listens for communication activity in the network. If the line is free, the computer sends its information. If not, the station waits and tries again later. In case two or more nodes attempt to transmit at the same time, resulting in a collision, the collision monitor in each station immediately cuts off the transmission. Since no one station dictates the transmission right, each station will compete again for the right to transmit after a random period of time. Each node will repeat the "listen, pause, or transmit" procedure until the line is free. The Ethernet, developed by Xerox, is the best known CSMA. Due to a collision problem, the average transmission rate in a busy Ethernet is limited to 500 KB/second instead of the rated top speed of 10 MB/second.

AN OVERVIEW OF PACS

Regardless of its many different components and its design sophistication, a PACs must be able to perform the following functions: acquire images in digital form into the computer network; store the acquired images; transmit and retrieve images to and from storage; process the images; and display images and text information. The specific requirements for each of these functions on a PACS varies, depending on the type of images it is designed to handle. For example, requirements for acquisition, communication, processing, and display of an x-ray computed tomography images are different from those of chest radiographs or nuclear medicine images. The remainder of this chapter will describe the performance requirements of a PACS in the nuclear medicine environment. Since the acquisition of radionuclide images from the gamma camera into the computer has been discussed thoroughly in the previous chapters, this requirement of a PACS will not be repeated here.

Image Display Station

One of the concerns facing physicians contemplating an all-digital imaging department is whether the video display will offer the same resolution as that of film. The answer to this concern lies in the size of the image matrix that can be displayed by the video monitor. Current video technology is quite capable of displaying an image that has been digitized to a 1024 x 1024 matrix. Since the resolution of a gamma camera is adequately represented by a 256 x 256 image matrix, the images can be displayed on any high-resolution video display monitor with no degradation in the image quality.

The more important consideration for a nuclear medicine display station is whether it has the ability to display simultaneously a number of images to enable the physician to perform comparative interpretation. In addition, the physician should be able to perform some simple image manipulation functions such as smoothing, zooming, and gray scale adjustment on the viewing console whenever necessary. Although the current technology can easily meet these requirements, the image display console is nevertheless a weak link in the current nuclear medicine viewing station. Commercial systems with multiple viewing monitors are available to display multiple sets of nuclear medicine images in static or cinematic mode for comparative viewing, as well as graphs, annotated patient histories and interpretation results. However, much software still needs to be developed, refined and integrated with the hardware before the physician can effectively utilize it as a diagnostic tool.

Digital Image Storage System

Due to the small image matrix that is sufficient for digitizing nuclear medicine images, current digital storage technology is well within the capability required by a nuclear medicine PACS. For example, Winchester disks with a storage capacity from 450 to 800 MB are a well-developed technology. Also, the physical dimensions of Winchester disks have been reduced so much in recent years that several of them can be mounted together in a storage device the size of a filing cabinet to provide several gigabytes of fast on-line storage. Winchester disk systems also can be used to store several months of radionuclide images and allows rapid access to physicians with a high degree of reliability. Images not requiring frequent access can be stored on magnetic tapes or optical disks. Thus, storage of radionuclide images in a nuclear medicine PACS is a manageable task; this is in contrast with the large volume of digital x-ray images that push current storage devices to their limit, especially since a solution still awaits advances in storage technology.

Patient Information Management

This is another aspect that PACS, whether they are nuclear medicine or radiology PACS, must improve. Current patient information management components of most PACS focus on indexing the whereabouts of patient images by name, patient file number, or study type. A useful nuclear medicine PACS should, however, incorporate the physician's interpretation report or patient history as an integral part of each patient's portfolio that can be displayed next to the images. The solution to this problem lies in integrating a reporting system with the PACS so that text and image information for each patient can be kept together in the computer just like a patient folder with film and dictation reports in the file room.

Problems With State-of-The-Art PACs

There are two major areas that state-of-the-art PACS must address and constantly improve. First, the software must be fun to use and not require extensive training. Otherwise, technologists would rather run to the darkroom to process films than send images through the computer network to the physician's display console. Likewise, the menu options on the control console must be self-explantory. If physicians have to struggle with the computer each and every time to bring up the desired images for viewing and interpretation, then they too would prefer to see the images on fluorescent light boxes and to flip through papers in the file folder for other clinical information.

Second, data communication speed has to improve. A few minutes may seem like a short time to send a set of images from an acquisition and processing node to a display node on a different floor. However, in a department with a number of acquisition and processing nodes, several minutes of transmission time for each set of images may create tremendous traffic congestion in the network. Solutions for the slowness of data communication will have to wait until the development of low-noise parallel transmission technology to replace the present serial transmission methods.

CONCLUSION

Computer networking is a natural progression as computers have become an inseparable part of the equipment for nuclear medicine studies. The modest amount of storage required for gamma camera images is advantageous for the development of a nuclear medicine PACS because one of the major stumbling blocks for PACS in radiology is finding ways to store the enormous amount of digital data generated from radiographic images. For example, a 14 x 17 chest radiograph when converted to digital form requires an image matrix of at least 1024 x 1024 and preferably 2048 x 2048 pixels in order to reproduce the original image resolution. These image matrices correspond to 1 MB and 4 MB of computer storage, respectively. As a comparison, between 16 to 1024 radionuclide images could fit in the space required to hold just one chest radiograph in the computer. Another factor for the use of nuclear medicine PACS is that there is no need to purchase special computer equipment for the sole purpose of converting analog gamma camera images into digital form. In most hospitals, one or more computers are already available in the department for performing routine gated cardiac blood-pool studies and emission tomography.

In spite of the difficulties experienced by the pioneering systems, the future for an all-digital nuclear medicine department is bright and inevitable. The experience we gain from developing and using nuclear medicine networks will no doubt provide valuable information for the development of other medical imaging network systems.

SUGGESTED READINGS

1. Apple Computers. *Understanding computer networks.* Addison-Wesley: Apple Computer, Inc., 1988.

2. Nunemacher G. *LAN Primer—an introduction to local area networks.* Redwood City, CA: M&T Books; 1990.

3. Perry JR, Thompson BG, Stabb EV, Pizer SM, Johnson RE. Performance features for a PACS display console. *Computer IEE Computer Society* 1983;16:51-56.

4. Thrall JH. Image communication and image analysis: meeting diagnostic radiologists' needs. Proceedings of the 1987 Amerian Association of Physicists in Medicine Summer School at University of Michigan, Ann Arbor, MI.

CHAPTER

11

CRITERIA FOR THE SELECTION OF A COMPUTER FOR NUCLEAR MEDICINE

INTRODUCTION

The selection of a nuclear medicine computer system is a complicated task for both novice and experienced users. Part of the problem is that the list of hardware, software, and other features essential for nuclear medicine is nearly identical for all vendors. However, if we take a close look at the vendor's specifications and consult with current users, we may realize that the efficacy with which the hardware and software are integrated into a system to address various clinical needs varies widely from one vendor to another. Therefore, the buyer must understand not only what the computer system will do, but also how competing systems perform. While the selection criteria and its relative importance will differ from institution to institution, there are many functional requirements common to all users. This chapter illustrates some of the factors that are important for a computer in the clinical nuclear medicine environment. Of course, the ensuing discussion should be treated only as one user's point of view. The prospective buyer should weigh the importance of these factors relative to his/her own needs and constraints.

The most important considerations for a nuclear medicine computer are the clinical application software that comes with the system and the service support offered by the manufacturer. However, software is also limited by the capability of its hardware. System reliability and the promptness of the field service to correct malfunctioning equipment are also important, especially for institutions located far away from the service center and for smaller departments with just one computer, where delays in equipment repair could severely hamper clinical operations.

SOFTWARE

A nuclear medicine computer system is only as good as the clinical application software provided to the user to perform diagnostic studies. All commercial systems list the ability to perform quantitative static and dynamic cardiac studies, curve analyses, common image manipulation functions, and SPECT. However, the accuracy, richness of features, flexibility, speed, and friendliness of the clinical software vary tremendously among systems. While some of the differences can be attributed to the different capabilities of the hardware, many of the differences are the consequences of the design structure of the software, the length of time the software has been in use clinically, and the resources of the vendor to continually refine their software and develop new applications. There are four areas in which software may have the greatest impact on how effectively the computer can be utilized for clinical studies: data acquisition, processing, user-friendliness, and display.

Data Acquisition Software

Relatively small differences are found among vendors in the sophistication of their hardware and software to acquire images from the gamma camera into the computer. With most computers, the radionuclide images are stored in the memory as a square matrix, typically of 64 x 64, 128 x 128, and 256 x 256 pixels; many newer computers on the market also provide acquisition matrices of 512 x 512 and 1024 x 1024. Since the maximum resolution of the state-of-the-art gamma camera with a 40-cm diameter field of view is adequately represented by a 256 x 256 matrix, there is no need to utilize a greater image matrix. In other words, using a 512 x 512 matrix to capture the image from a gamma camera with a 40-cm diameter crystal will not improve image resolution because the ultimate resolution of the image on the computer is limited by the resolution of the gamma camera, not the matrix size. However, owners of jumbo-size gamma cameras with a crystal dimension greater than 40 cm will find it necessary to acquire images in 512 x 512 or even 1024 x 1024 matrix. Also, users with a gamma camera having a rectangular field of view will find the image presented in a square matrix appears compressed in one direction and elongated in the perpendicular direction. Some vendors have addressed this problem by providing rectangular matrices such as 64 x 128, 128 x 256, and 256 x 512 to acquire images from a rectangular field of view camera or total-body scans.

It is desirable and at times absolutely necessary that the software allows the user to separate the acquisition of a flow study into two or more phases, each with its own set of acquisition parameters. The program should give the user the option to specify the desired acquisition time per frame, the number of frames, delay time between two consecutive frames in each phase, and also the time interval between two phases. The acquisition parameters for each phase should be defined beforehand so that there is no need to pause while the user changes the acquisition parameters between two phases and, thereby miss flow information. Unfortunately, not all commercial software are able to provide this flexibility for dynamic acquisitions.

The framing rate and the number of frames that the computer can acquire without pauses depend strongly on the speed of the hardware and the amount of memory in the system. Most of the systems on the market today have 1 MB to 2 MB of video display memory, which is also used for storing the data during acquisition. Some newer systems have up to 8 MB of memory dedicated for image display and acquisition, while a few systems still utilize 512 KB or less. Systems with a limited amount of memory will have to halt acquisition periodically to transfer data from the memory to the disk, resulting in a loss of counts during the time of transfer.

One of the performance criteria we often overlook is the rate at which the computer can acquire counts from the gamma camera without losses. We unquestioningly assume that the computer is able to acquire data at least as fast as the gamma camera. However, some users have reported that at count rates as low as 10,000 cps their gamma camera could acquire data faster than it could be converted by the computer; one of the computers used by the author became completely paralyzed at about 50,000 cps. The only way to reactivate the computer was by shutting the power off and then on again to reboot. As a minimum requirement, the computer must be able to acquire 50,000 cps without any losses in order to meet the needs of first-pass cardiac studies, and preferrably up to 100,000 cps for users of high-speed gamma cameras and short-lived radionuclides. We can easily assess the count rate capability of the computer by acquiring an intrinsic flood image of a ^{99m}Tc source of 300 mCi for 10 seconds at various distances from the crystal. At each counting rate, the number of counts acquired into the image matrix should match the number of counts shown on the camera console to within 1% of each other. On some integrated camera-computer systems, the user may not be able to obtain the image matrix counts separate from the gamma camera counts. For these systems, the user could acquire a series of images with sources of different activity at a fixed distance from the crystal. A plot of the number of counts in the image matrix versus the activity in the source should follow a straight line. The analysis of the resulting curve becomes complicated at the high count rate region as the deviation of the curve from a straight line result from both the dropoff of the counting rate of the gamma camera and the computer. The count versus activity curve is thus an indication of the overall count rate capability of the camera-computer system, not just the camera or computer alone.

The requirements for radionuclide blood-pool studies were discussed at length in Chapter 8. In summary, the software for gated blood-pool studies must provide the means to reject a bad beat. The user should be able to select the number of frames to store the data for one complete cardiac cycle. For example, the user should have the freedom to acquire data from a patient into 16 frames to obtain good count statistics for cine display or into 32 or more frames to obtain good temporal resolution for curve analyses.

List-mode acquisition is an outdated method. Given today's high-speed processors and inexpensive memory, the rate of data acquisition should be limited by the counting rate of the gamma camera, not the computer, (i.e., a modern computer should be able to acquire high counting rate studies, such as the cardiac first-pass study, using the frame acquisition method with no loss of data). Currently, all nuclear medicine computers still offer list-mode acquisition as an obligatory feature, but the software is infrequently updated and much too cumbersome for reformatting data into image frames.

Processing Software

Since the user will spend the most time working with processing software, it should be given the most consideration at the time of equipment selection. The concern with processing software lies not in whether some systems can perform certain image processing functions than competing systems, but in the friendliness of the user interface, and the efficiency with which the software is integrated with the hardware. The industry has matured to the point that every commercial nuclear medicine system on the market offers nearly the same processing capabilities.

Processing software consists of a collection of programs for the enhancement and quantitative analysis of the acquired images. Some programs are linked together in a predefined sequence to form a clinical protocol, such as the protocols for the calculation of glomerular filtration rate, cardiac ejection fraction, pulmonary ventilation/perfusion ratio, and tomographic image reconstruction.

Clinical processing protocols are indispensible because they provide a well-defined processing procedure for each clinical study so that follow-up patient studies can be processed consistently. In order to produce consistent results, however, the predefined protocols should carry out its processing functions automatically with only little user input initially. Predefined protocols also expedite the processing by bringing up the processing steps automatically one after another. Unfortunately, some clinical protocols require a rigid data structure. Frequently due to the patient conditions or user mistakes, the data could not be acquired with the exact image sequence, matrix size, patient positions, or the number of images as specified by the protocol. A well thought out program would allow the user the means for adapting predefined protocols to fit the clinical data at hand or making adjustments on the patient data to fit the processing procedure. It is all too common to find that many pre-packaged clinical programs are just too difficult for the user to adjust the processing procedure or data format to fit certain patient study protocols. Furthermore, some vendor's software show little changes year after year in spite of repeated user complaints. These problems are symptomatic of software designed originally with such a rigid structure that any modification may require extensive changes that the vendor is reluctant to make. A worse scenario may be that the manufacturer is unable to make software changes due to limitations of the hardware.

USER SUPPORT

Regardless of how user-friendly the software may be, users will still have questions from time to time on how to use certain features of the software. They will discover software bugs and will have needs not met by the current software. Of course, the finite resources of the manufacturer will not be able to fulfill all of the demands of its large number of customers. However, the manufacturer should provide readily available personnel to answer questions from the novice to the sophisticated users. Most major vendors provide an application specialist to give initial training to the new users and to make periodic follow-up visits for solving common problems.

Although the algorithms and image processing principles are well known and can be easily found in the literature, some vendors maintain an archaic policy of not releasing the source codes to general users. In order to customize pre-packaged software or to develop new routines not available in the supplied software package, the user needs access to the source codes and assistance from the vendor on the utilization of the software library. These buyers could specify in the contract that the vendor makes available the source codes along with the associated documents upon request as a condition of purchase. The buyer should also carefully evaluate the vendor's attitude in helping present users to program on their computer systems.

No matter how long the software has been in development and in use clinically, there are always bugs to be corrected and improvements to be made. Also, in the purchase of a nuclear medicine computer system, most of the cost is in the software, not the hardware. Therefore, vendors should provide software updates to the users with no more than a nominal charge to defray the handling expenses.

Equally important is that the manufacturer makes serious efforts to resolve difficulties encountered by users and to incorporate user suggestions into their new software releases. The responsiveness of the manufacturers to the needs of the users can be judged by the resources and commitment of the manufacturer to the ongoing development of its software and hardware. Site visits and discussions with current users will help the buyer assess these qualities.

MEASUREMENT OF USER FRIENDLINESS

Although user-friendliness is a subjective assessment, we can judge the ease with which the user can utilize the computer in terms of several factors. For example, we could compare the degree of forgiveness to user input errors. During the input of information to the computer, we will invariably make typing errors, change our mind after a making a menu selection, or need to modify parts of the region of interest after it has been drawn. A user-friendly program would allow the user to make these changes rapidly without having to repeat a number of other input steps. A user-hostile system is one that ignores the pleads of the user for an opportunity to correct one's mistakes. In such a circumstance, the user has no choice but to let the computer processing continue with the undesired input until it is done or "bombs out." In another scenario, the lack of error checking in the software could cause the system to freeze and force the infuriated user to restart the system by turning the power off and then on again.

User-friendliness can also be measured by the amount of human interaction required to initiate and complete a given processing function. Much of the computer and operator dialogue can be eliminated if the software is designed so that information already present in various parts of the program did not have to be re-entered.

In the name of user-friendliness, all commercial nuclear medicine computers make use of menus as a means of interaction between the user and the computer. However, not all menus were created equally friendly. To be useful, the meanings behind the menu options must be obvious and there should be enough exit branches for the user to move from one type of operation to another without erasing the intermediate result in memory. A poorly designed menu is frustrating because the user could get trapped in a menu page and not know how to exit except by powering down the system. A menu full of incomprehensive mnemonics is worse than having no menu at all because it forces the user to guess the meaning of the selection. Often, a wrong guess could cause the user to lose everything that the computer has computed up to that point.

IMAGE DISPLAY

The quality of the image display system is a function of the video display hardware and the software used to manipulate the presentation of the images on the screen. A traditional display system uses a single color or gray scale to show images on a video monitor with a 256 x 256 pixel resolution so that one 256 x 256, four 128 x 128, or sixteen 64 x 64 images can be shown simultaneously. Two problems exist with this type of display. If the patient study has more images than can be shown on-screen at any one time, the images will have to be viewed in sequence, one screen after another. This makes comparative interpretation of the images difficult, especially if the study is acquired as a follow-up study or is acquired dynamically with many images. With the decreasing cost of high-resolution video monitors, computer memory and high-speed graphic processors, monitors that can display 1024 x 1024 pixels are fast becoming the standard for nuclear medicine computer systems. When using a 1024 x 1024 resolution display monitor, sixteen times as many images can be shown on the screen simultaneously. There are still more sophisticted systems that can display images simultaneously on two or more 1024 x 1024 resolution monitors. However, these multiple display systems are presently marketed as a separate display station, rather than as a part of the nuclear medicine computer.

The newer computer systems can also support several simultaneous color or gray scales so that images, such as bone and liver scans with widely different count densities, can be adjusted individually for side-by-side viewing on the screen at optimal viewing intensities and color scales.

In addition to image quality, we should also examine how easily we can select images from one or more studies of the same patient for comparative interpretation. Although all nuclear medicine computers allow the user to perform image manipulation functions such as smoothing or contrast enhancement, the amount of labor involved varies considerably. Some systems allow the user to process selected images on-screen without disturbing the other images, while other systems require the user to exit from the display routine in order to work on the desired images and then recompose the screen for interpretation. These variations on system performance again reflect the efficiency and flexibility of the software and hardware integration.

HARDWARE

In the evaluation of the system hardware, we can become preoccupied with comparing the speed of the central processing unit (CPU), memory size, the amount of disk storage, etc. and lose sight of the fact that the hardware is only as good as its software. With the stabilization of many hardware and system software as the de facto standards of the computer industry, we may see that many nuclear medicine systems are using hardware from the same computer equipment manufacturers. The distinction between competing nuclear medicine systems is more in the efficiency of integrated hardware and software to form a useful clinical tool than in the muscle power of each individual computer component. For example, a system designed to perform at or near capacity does not allow for future addition of peripheral equipment or expansion of the software capability. Manufacturers may also build limitations or make modifications of the standard hardware to make their product unique and to inhibit other vendors from attaching their equipment to the system. Therefore, we should evaluate the hardware in terms of the potentials and limitations that the hardware may present to future expansion of the system and developments of new clinical software. One of the hardware components that has the strongest influence on software development is the CPU. After a decade of evolution, the CPU of choice has moved from the 16-bit mini-computers to the 16-bit microprocessors and is now migrating toward the 32-bit version. With the faster execution speed of the 32-bit CPU and the assistance of a numeric co-processor, many computation-intense tasks such as tomographic image reconstruction can be done without the array processor. The next generation of software with the ability to do concurrent processing, artificial intelligence, and three-dimensional imaging, is being developed to run on these 32-bit processors. Therefore, systems built on the 32-bit processors will be able to offer new application software not practical on the current 16-bit systems. However, for routine tasks in nuclear medicine, the 16-bit processors serve the purpose admirably well.

The amount of CPU memory is always quoted in every system proposal. However, the user rarely, if at all, has a choice to purchase more or less than the quoted amount of memory because this parameter is fixed for a given system at the time of its design. One can make a mild inference, however, that the processing speed and the sophistication of the software generally is proportional to the amount of CPU memory supported by the system.

No user will ever regret selecting the largest and fastest disk storage device that the computer system and their budget allow. High capacity disk drives are indispensible for all nuclear medicine systems, especially those used for emission tomography. Since images require a large amount of computer storage, a high capacity disk offers the user the convenience of storing a large number of patient images on-line, which can be retrieved rapidly for processing or viewing. Fortunately, the high-performance Winchester disk, once regarded as an expensive option for the elites, keeps increasing its storage capacity and reliability and decreasing its physical size and cost.

No matter how large the disk capacity may be, it will always be filled much sooner than the user had expected. Therefore, each system should have at least one backup device such as a tape drive an optical disk drive, or even a floppy disk drive to unload older data from the disk in order to make room for new patient data. The data recorded on the off-line media also becomes a part of the patient's records in the department and can be retrieved later for reprocessing or review when necessary.

Display is one of the most important features of any image processing system. Unfortunately, the makers of nuclear medicine computers have neglected display until recently, when they realized that this was an area in which they could improve to distinguish their system from that of their competitors. As is the case for CPU and memory, there are few options for the user in choosing the type of display hardware for a given system. Most nuclear medicine computers designed in the 1970s and 1980s utilize two monitors on their display system, one for the display of text and menu options, and the other to display the images. State-of-the-art computers with graphical user interface (GUI), tear-off menus, and pop-up windows utilize one large monitor of about 19 inches in diameter for both text and image display.

One must keep in mind that image resolution depends on the number of pixels that the data are stored in, and not the size of the display screen. In fact, the sharpness of an image decreases as the size of the screen increases because the same number of image pixels is spread over a larger area. A video monitor of about 13 inches diagonally appears to be optimum for the display of radionuclide images in a 256 x 256 pixel matrix. For systems that could display larger matrices, such as 512 x 512 or 1024 x 1024, the screen should be proportionately bigger so that the images will not become too small at the normal viewing distance.

RELIABILITY AND SERVICE SUPPORT

Reliability and service support are basic concerns because frequent breakdowns can severely erode the confidence of referring physicians, the acceptance of the system by the user, and ultimately its utilization for clinical diagnosis. System uptime is directly related to its reliability, which begins with the system design and extends through all facets of engineering, sales, and service. Good engineering design assures system reliability by integrating industry-proven hardware and standard "system software" into a readily serviceable and expandable system. The buyer should consult with colleagues knowledgeable about computers if he is unable to judge the reliability of the system's design. The buyer should also request that the sales representative disclose any components not in the vendor's usual product line but included in the proposed system in order to meet specifications; this is an important piece of information because any new or non-standard components that have not undergone thorough testing could severely affect the system reliability.

System reliability and the quality of service suport can be judged by consulting current users of the system. The pertinent data to obtain from these users include: frequency of system breakdown, response time to the service call, waiting time for any parts not in stock, and the thoroughness of the repair service. Finally, the buyer should find out the length of the warranty period and whether the usual service contract includes all parts, regularly scheduled preventive maintenance, corrective maintenance, and a guaranteed service response time.

CONCLUSION

The selection of a computer system for nuclear medicine is the result of a compromise between the needs of the user and what is available on the market. It may be a difficult proposition, but the selection process will become a little easier if the nuclear medicine community could develop a test protocol for benchmarking the relative performance of nuclear medicine computer systems.

The selection criteria discussed in this chapter reflect some of the problems that I encountered from using several commercially available computers. There are many other evaluation criteria such as those related to SPECT, vendor viability, package deals with a gamma camera, etc. that have not been discussed. The buyer should make up a list of specific performance criteria and then evaluate the computer configurations proposed to him in terms of the outlined needs. Consultation with existing users with nearly the same proposed configuration and the same type of clinical operations are most valuable in reaffirming the sales presentations and perhaps refining the buyer's list of selection criteria. Do not assume anything. The vendor's denotation may not be your connotation of the terms. Ask questions no matter how trivial they may seem and seek answers in a manner understandable to both the purchaser and the manufacturer. Never forget to put in writing the specifications that you feel are essential for your clinical needs.

One last piece of advice: avoid buying computers at the end of the manufacturer's product cycle for the simple reason that computer technology advances at a dizzying pace. Even the latest computer model will be hard pressed to run software designed for computers to be released next year. Therefore, buying aged computers will only accelerate the obsolescence rate of department equipment. On the other hand, the buyer should not be lured by promises of the future into purchasing *vaporware*. Vaporware is the highly touted new and wonderful hardware or software of the future that can be purchased today, but has no chance of performing to the specifications or of even being delivered by the manufacturer. When presented with such a dilemma, potential buyers should consult knowledgeable users on the likelihood of "to be released" products performing as advertised.

SUGGESTED READING

1. Graham MM, Links JM, Lewellen TK, et al. Considerations in the purchase of a nuclear medicine computer system. *J Nucl Med* 1988;29:717-724.

APPENDIX

DIGITAL NUMBER SYSTEMS

The Decimal System

The decimal system uses a positional value notation to represent numbers. Using the positional value system, the value of a digit is weighted by its position relative to the decimal point. Consider the number 191. Although the digit 1 on the left hand side of the 9 is identical to the 1 on the right, these two digits represent very different quantities. The meaning of 191 becomes evident when we speak of it as one hundred and ninety one. The first digit 1 on the left hand side actually represents one hundred, the 9 represents nine tens, and the last digit 1 represents one. Therefore, the number 191 is equivalent to:

(1 x 100) + (9 x 10) + 1.

The following example illustrates that the positional multiplier of a digit equals to 10 raised to the nth power, where n is the number of places the digit is away from the decimal point. The value of the entire number is calculated as the sum of the products of each digit times its positional multiplier.

Multiplier	10^4	10^3	10^2	10^1	10^0	.	10^{-1}	10^{-2}	10^{-3}
Digit	0	0	1	9	1	.	0	0	0
191	=0	+0	+1×10^2	+9×10^1	+1×10^0	.	0	+0	+0

Decimal Counting

The radix of a number system is the number of different symbols or digits that can be used in each position. The digit 9 is the largest of the ten possible digits (0...9) that can occur in any given position in a number. After reaching 9, 0 is recycled back into that position and the next higher digital position is increased by 1. For n number of digital positions, the highest numerical value that can occur is $10^n - 1$. When given five positions to display a number, the highest numerical value that can be displayed is

$$9\quad 9\quad 9\quad 9\quad 9$$

(exactly what I saw on my car's odometer a few years back). However, with five digits, 10^5 different numbers can be expressed because we can count from 0 to 99,999 which gives us 100,000 different numbers. Therefore, the number of combinations representable by n digits, including zero, is equal to the radix raised to the nth power, but the highest numerical value is equal to the radix raised to the nth power - 1.

The Binary System

The binary system also uses the positional value notation to represent numbers. All of the rules described for the decimal system also apply to the binary system. Unlike the decimal system, the binary system has only two symbols for digits, 0 and 1. Any quantity that can be expressed in the decimal system can be expressed in the binary system, except that more binary digits may be required to represent the same numerical quantity. The positional multiplier of a binary digit or bit is expressed as 2 raised to a power equal to the number of places that the digit is displaced from the binary point. In other words, the positional multiplier of a bit is equal to 2^n, where n is the number of places the digit is displaced from the binary point. Bits lying to the left of the binary point are given positional multipliers which are positive powers of 2, while bits to the right of the binary point are negative powers of 2 as in the following diagram:

$$2^3\quad 2^2\quad 2^1\quad 2^0\quad \bullet\quad 2^{-1}\quad 2^{-2}\quad 2^{-3}$$

APPENDIX A 257

Using this information, we can convert any number in the binary form to the more familiar decimal form. For the following binary number: 1 0 1 1 1 1 1 1, converting the above number in the binary form to its decimal equivalent is simple. All it takes is adding together the positional multipliers of bits that carry a 1:

Multiplier 2^7 2^6 2^5 2^4 2^3 2^2 2^1 2^0

Binary   1   0   1   1   1   1   1   1

128 + 0 + 32 + 16 + 8 + 4 + 2 + 1 = 191

A binary number containing a fractional part can be converted to its decimal equivalent using the same method. For example, the binary number 101.101 is converted to its decimal equivalent as follows:

Multiplier 2^2 2^1 2^0 . 2^{-1} 2^{-2} 2^{-3}

Binary   1   0   1   .   1   0   1

Decimal 1×2^2 + 0 + 1×2^0 . 1×2^{-1} + 0 + 1×2^{-3} = 5.625

Decimal to Binary Conversion

The conversion is done in two stages. The first stage converts the integers, the portion of the number to the left of the decimal point; the second stage converts the fractional part of the number to the right of the decimal point. Let us convert the number 18.373 to binary as an illustration. Conversion of the integer 18 is done by repeatedly dividing it by 2, writing down the remainder after each division, and continuing on until a quotient of zero is obtained:

18/2 = 9 + remainder of 0
9/2 = 4 + 1
4/2 = 2 + 0
2/2 = 1 + 0
1/2 = 0 + 1

18 = 1 0 0 1 0

Thus, the decimal number 18 is equivalent to the binary number 1 0 0 1 0. Note that the first remainder is closest to the binary point, while the last remainder is farthest from the binary point.

The only difference between converting fraction and whole numbers is that they are multiplied instead of divided as above. In other words, the decimal fraction is converted to binary notation by multiplying the decimal fraction by 2 and recording any carries into the integer position. The process is continued until we get a zero remainder. Using this method to convert the decimal fraction to binary fraction, we get

0.375 x 2 = 0.750 = 0.750   carry   0

0.750 x 2 = 1.50 = 0.50   carry   1

0.50 x 2 = 1.00 = 0.00   carry   1

0.375 = 0. 0 1 1

Again, the first carry over into the integer position is written closest to the right of the binary point. It should be emphasized that we rarely obtain an even product 1.00 with a zero remainder. The process is usually forced to terminate after a predetermined number of bits is used, which is one of the reasons why analog-to-digital converters with a greater number of bits usually give a higher conversion precision.

APPENDIX

B

SUCCESSIVE APPROXIMATION ADC: HOW IT WORKS

The successive approximation method is explained by showing the steps taken by an ADC to convert an analog signal representing the x-coordinate of a count from the gamma camera to the binary form. Readers not familiar with the binary number system are urged to review Appendix A before continuing with the following discussion. The successive approximation method is a trial and error procedure. The process starts by flipping on the most significant bit. The bit is turned off if the binary value represented by the high-bit binary number is greater than the input value, and is left on if it is less. The next bit is turned on to compare the sum total of the binary digits with the input value. The second bit is left on if the binary total is less than the input and turned off if the binary total is greater. This same comparison procedure is repeated for each bit until the least significant bit is checked. After the comparison of the least significant bit is completed, the final string of ones and zeroes becomes the output digital number.

To illustrate the above description, let us use an ADC that has six bits to hold the output result. The biggest numerical value that the ADC can hold is $2^6 - 1$ or 63. Assume that the incoming analog signal has a numerical value of 25. Referring to Figure B-1, the following steps will be taken by the ADC to convert the analog signal to the digital form.

1. At the start all the bits are set to zero.
2. The most significant bit, Bit A, is turned on to give a value of 32.

3. Since 32 is greater than 25, Bit A is turned off and Bit B is turned on. Since Bit B represents 16 and is lower than 25, Bit B is left on.
4. Bit C, representing 8, is then turned on. Together Bit B and Bit C give a sum of 24 and this is still lower than 25; so Bit C stays on.
5. When Bit D, representing 4, is turned on, the sum total becomes 28 and is greater than 25;
6. Bit D is turned off, and Bit E, representing 2, is flipped on next, the binary sum of Bits B, C, E equals to 26 and is greater than 25.
7. So Bit E is turned off. Bit F, representing 1, is flipped on. The binary sum of Bits B, C, and F becomes equal to but not greater than 25. Hence Bit F is left on. At the end we have a 6-bit digital signal equal to 011001 going to the computer.

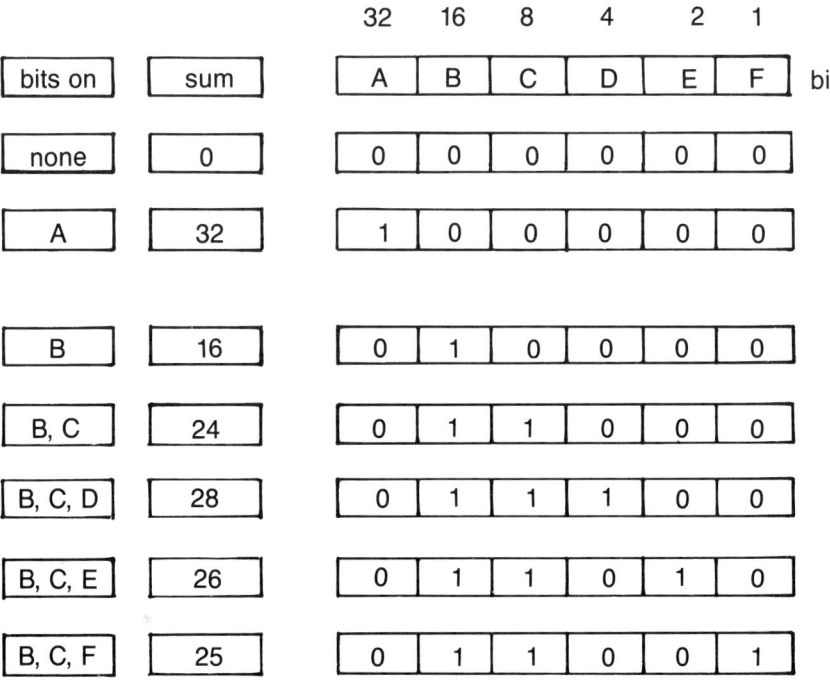

FIGURE B-1 Successive approximation.

APPENDIX B

As you can see from the example, if the input is 100, the input signal must be scaled down. Otherwise, the 6-bit ADC will not be able to represent the analog signal adequately. Therefore, the maximum input signal and the precision with which an input value can be processed by the ADC is directly proportional to the number of bits used by the ADC. Since the resolution of a gamma camera is adequately represented by an array of 256 x 256 pixels, the x- and y-coordinates of a gamma camera event can be adequately handled by two 8-bit ADC (2^8 = 256). For high-precision measurements, however, ADCs with 12-20 bits are invariably used to convert the magnitude of an analog signal to the binary form.

There are four other parameters in addition to the number of bits used to characterize the performance of an ADC: conversion speed, resolution, linearity, and quantizing error. More ambitious readers are referred to the literature for more in-depth discussion, because even a cursory discussion of these parameters will involve engineering "nitty gritty" that will bore the majority of my readers.

APPENDIX

C

FOURIER TRANSFORM

The concept of Fourier transform was explained in detail in Chapter 6. The computational procedure is explained in three sample functions. To show that Fourier transform is actually quite simple, I will not give any proof or try to be exact for the mathematical statements in the following examples.

When using the computer to perform Fourier transform on a sequence of numbers, such as $x_0, x_1, x_2, x_3, \ldots x_{N-1}$, we use a method known as the *discrete Fourier transform* (DFT), which approximates the continuous Fourier integral with the following two sets of finite summations:

$$RE_j = \sum_{i=0}^{N-1} x_i \cos(2\,i\,j/N),$$

$$IM_j = -\sum_{i=0}^{N-1} x_i \sin(2\,i\,j/N),$$

where

i is the sequential order of the ordinary variable x,
i = 0, 1, 2, . . .N-1
j represents the frequency harmonic, j = 0, 1, . . .N-1-
N is the total number of data points in the sequence.

RE_j is the discrete cosine Fourier transform of x_i in harmonic j, and IM_j is the discrete sine Fourier transform of x_i in harmonic j, respectively. In complex algebra terminology RE_j is called the real, and IM_j the imaginary, terms of the Fourier transform. When j = 0, $RE_{j=0}$ and $IM_{j=0}$ represent the DC components of transform, and the first harmonic $RE_{j=1}$ and $IM_{j=1}$ describe the fundamental frequency. The magnitude of the Fourier transform at each frequency harmonic is calculated by:

$$M_j = (RE_j^2 + IM_j^2)^{1/2}.$$

The phase angle is defined as that angle whose tangent is given by the ratio IM_j/RE_j: i.e.

$$\text{phase angle} = (180/\pi) \tan^{-1} (IM_j/RE_j).$$

Example 1

Perform Fourier transform on the following sequence of consecutive numbers, and calculate the magnitude and phase angle of the first harmonic.

$$x_j = 10, 20, 30, 40$$

Solution

Real terms are computed using Equation C-1 as follows:

$$RE_j = \sum_{i=0}^{N-1} x_i \cos(2\pi i j/N)$$

where i = 0, 1, 2, 3;   j = 0, 1, 2, 3;   and N = 4

$RE_{j=0}$ = 10 cos (2π0·0/4) + 20 cos (2π1·0/4) + 30 cos (2π2·0/4) + 40 cos (2π3·0/4)
= 10 + 20 + 30 + 40
= 100

$RE_{j=1}$ = 10 cos (2π0·1/4) + 20 cos (2π1·1/4) + 30 cos (2π2·1/4) + 40 cos (2π3·1/4)
= 10 + 0 + −30 + 0
= −20

APPENDIX C 265

$$RE_{j=2} = 10 \cos(2\pi 0 \cdot 2/4) + 20 \cos(2\pi 1 \cdot 2/4) + 30 \cos(2\pi 2 \cdot 2/4) + \\ 40 \cos(2\pi 3 \cdot 2/4)$$
$$= 10 + -20 + 30 + -40$$
$$= -20$$

$$RE_{j=3} = 10 \cos(2\pi 0 \cdot 3/4) + 20 \cos(2\pi 1 \cdot 3/4) + 30 \cos(2\pi 2 \cdot 3/4) + \\ 40 \cos(2\pi 3 \cdot 3/4)$$
$$= 10 + 0 + -30 + 0$$
$$= -20$$

The imaginary terms are computed using Equation C-2 as follows:

$$IM_j = \sum_{i=0}^{N-1} x_i \sin(2\pi i j/N),$$

$$IM_{j=0} = -[10 \sin(2\pi 0 \cdot 0/4) + 20 \sin(2\pi 1 \cdot 0/4) + 30 \sin(2\pi 2 \cdot 0/4) + \\ 40 \sin(2\pi 3 \cdot 0/4)]$$
$$= -[0 + 0 + 0 + 0]$$
$$= 0$$

$$IM_{j=1} = -[10 \sin(2\pi 0 \cdot 1/4) + 20 \sin(2\pi 1 \cdot 1/4) + 30 \sin(2\pi 2 \cdot 1/4) + \\ 40 \sin(2\pi 3 \cdot 1/4)]$$
$$= -[0 + 20 + -40]$$
$$= -20$$

$$IM_{j=2} = -[10 \sin(2\pi 0 \cdot 2/4) + 20 \sin(2\pi 1 \cdot 2/4) + 30 \sin(2\pi 2 \cdot 2/4) + \\ 40 \sin(2\pi 3 \cdot 2/4)]$$
$$-[0 + 0 + 0 + 0]$$
$$= 0$$

$$IM_{j=3} = -[10 \sin(2\pi 0 \cdot 3/4) + 20 \sin(2\pi 1 \cdot 3/4) + 30 \sin(2\pi 2 \cdot 3/4) + \\ 40 \sin(2\pi 3 \cdot 3/4)]$$
$$= -[0 + -20 + 0 + 40]$$
$$= -20$$

As a result of the above computations, we get

$$RE_j = 100, -20, -20, -20$$
$$IM_j = 0, 20, 0, -20.$$

The magnitude of the first harmonic is calculated as the square root of the sum of the squares of the real and imaginary components:

$$\begin{aligned}\text{magnitude} &= \sqrt{(RE_{j=1})^2 + (IM_{j=1})^2} \\ &= \sqrt{(-20)^2 + (20)^2} \\ &= 28.3\end{aligned}$$

The phase angle of the first harmonic is calculated as the arc-tangent of the ratio:

$$\frac{IM_{j=1}}{RE_{j=1}}$$

$$\begin{aligned}\text{phase} &= 180/\pi) \tan^{-1}(IM_{j=1}/RE_{j=1}) \\ &= (180/3.14159) \tan^{-1}[20/(-20)] \\ &= 135 \text{ degrees}\end{aligned}$$

Now that we have computed the Fourier transform, let us do an inverse transform to see if we can regenerate the original ordinary data. The inverse Fourier transform is performed using the following operation on the real and imaginary Fourier components:

$$x_j = (1/N) \left[\sum_{i=0}^{N-1} RE_j \cos(2\pi i\, j/N) + \sum_{i=0}^{N-1} IM_j \sin(2\pi i\, j/N) \right]$$

For the sake of brevity, let us only do the inverse Fourier transform of the last data point to see if we get 40 as the answer.

$$\begin{aligned}x_{j=3} =\ &(1/4\ [100 \cos (2\pi 3\ 0/4) + 0 \sin (2\pi 3\cdot 0/4) + \\ &-20 \cos (2\pi 3\ 1/4) + 20 \sin (2\pi 3\cdot 1/4) + \\ &-20 \cos (2\pi 3\ 2/4) + 0 \sin (2\pi 3\cdot 2/4) + \\ &-20 \cos (2\pi 3\ 3/4) + (-20)\sin (2\pi 3\cdot 3/4) + \\ =\ &(1/4)\ [100 + 0 + 20 + 0 + 20 + 0 + 0 + 20] \\ =\ &40\end{aligned}$$

APPENDIX C

The above example shows that DFT is straight-forward but requires a lot of repetitive computations. Without the computer, DFT by hand calculations is practical only up to 5 or 6 data points. For that reason, I wrote a short computer program as shown in Figure C-1 to do the Fourier transform for the next example.

Example 2

Given the two cosine functions shown as Curves A and B in Figure C-2, when Curve A is at its maximum, Curve B is at its minimum and vice versa, much like the volume curves for the ventricles and atria. Compute the DFT and the magnitude and phase of the first harmonic for both curves.

Solution

Using the computer program in Figure C-1, the DFT as well as the magnitude and phase of the two curves are computed and tabulated in Table C-1. For a curve of 13 points, the computation time is tolerable. For curves with more data points, such as 64 and 128 points in an emission computed tomography projection profile, the computation time becomes so long that we need to use a variation of the DFT called the fast Fourier transform (FFT) to do the computations on the computer, perhaps with an array processor.

Let us analyze the first harmonics of the DFT of Curves A and B by plotting the data in Table C-1 in a *phase diagram* as shown in Figure C-2. There Curves A and B are represented as two vectors in a cos versus sin plot. The two Vectors A and B have equal magnitude but are pointing in opposite directions, i.e., 180° apart. The result is exactly as expected because as Curve A rises to a maximum, Curve B decreases to a minimum, and vice versa.

The phase diagram also points out a *bug* in the simple computer program in Figure C-1 and a word of caution on the use of Equation C-4 to calculate the phase angle. The numerical value of the tangent of an angle is positive and identical in quadrants I and III, and is negative and identical in quadrants II and IV. The computer program assigned the same phase angle to both Curves A and B because it applied Equation C-4 to calculate the phase angle whose tangent is given by the ratio of the imaginary to the real components without consideration for the signs of the sine and cosine components. Readers may debug the computer program by adding a short algorithm to compute the phase angle in accordance with the signs of the real and imaginary components.

TABLE C-1

Harmonic	Cosine transform	Sine transform	Amplitude	Phase
Fourier Transform of Curve A				
0	1000.00	0.00	1000.00	0.00
1	6500.04	1602.13	6694.58	13.85
2	-352.53	-185.02	398.13	27.69
3	-100.67	-89.19	134.50	41.54
4	-35.40	-51.28	62.31	55.39
5	-10.41	-27.46	29.37	69.23
6	-1.07	-8.79	8.85	83.08
7	-1.06	-8.75	8.82	-83.08
8	-10.40	27.42	29.33	-69.23
9	-35.37	51.25	62.27	-55.38
10	-100.63	89.25	134.44	-41.54
11	-352.45	184.97	398.04	-27.69
12	6500.14	-1601.94	6694.63	-13.84
Fourier Transform of Curve B				
0	-999.98	0.00	999.98	0.00
1	-6500.05	602.13	6694.58	13.85
2	352.51	185.01	398.11	27.69
3	100.69	89.20	134.52	41.54
4	35.42	51.31	62.35	55.39
5	10.41	27.44	29.35	69.23
6	1.06	8.76	8.82	83.08
7	1.06	-8.72	8.79	-83.08
8	10.39	-27.40	29.31	-69.23
9	35.39	-51.28	62.31	-55.38
10	100.64	-89.16	134.46	-41.54
11	352.42	-184.95	398.00	-27.69
12	-6500.15	1601.94	6694.63	-13.84

APPENDIX C

```c
/*      This program was written using Microsoft Quick C 1.5      */
/*      to run on an IBM PC . The program was designed to show    */
/ *     the steps in the Fourier transform of an arbitrary function */
/ *     and was not optimized for speed or user friendliness!      */

#include <math.h>
#include <stdio.h>
#define twopi    6.28318
#define pi       3.14159

main()

{
        float      f[50], RE[50], IM[50], inverse, amplitude, phase;
        int        i, j, N;
        char       go;
/*      Section of code for user to enter data                  */

        printf ("\x1B[2J");     /*  clear screen for data entry */

        printf ("Enter number of data points : ");
        scanf ("%d", &N);

        for (i=0; i < N; i++)
          {
            printf ("\nEnter point %d:  ", i+1);
            scanf ("%f", &f[i]);
          }
/*      Clear screen and print headings */
        printf   ("\x1B[2J");
        printf ("                    Cosine           Sine\n");
        printf ("Harmonic       Transform        Transform       Amplitude
                   phase\n\n");

/*      RE is the real or cosine Fourier transform, IM is the imaginary  */
/*      or sine Fourier transform, J is the harmonic                    */

        for ( j=0; j < N; j++)
        {
          RE[j] = 0;
          IM[j] = 0;
          for ( i=0; i < N; i++)
          {
            RE[j] += f[i]*cos (twopi*i*j/N);
            IM[j] += f[i]*sin (twopi*i*j/N);
          }
          amplitude = sqrt ( RE[j]*RE[j] + IM[j]*IM[j]);

          phase     = (180.0/pi)* atan (-IM [j]/RE[j] );
          printf ("%5d  %12.2f    %14.2f  %12.2f   %12.2f\n",
                  j,  RE[j],    -IM[j], amplitude, phase);
        }

        printf ("\n\nHit any key to continue");
        go = getch();
        printf   ("\x1B[2J");
```

```
/*      Let us perform the inverse Fourier Transform here        */
/*     to regain the original data                       */

      printf ("Point    Original  data\n\n");
      for (i=0; i < N; i++)
      {
        inverse = 0;
        for (j=0; j < N; j++)
        {
            inverse  +=  RE[j]*cos(twopi*i*j/N)  +  IM[j]*sin(twopi*i*j/N);
        }
        inverse /= N;
        printf ("%3d     %8.2f\n", i+1, inverse);
      }
} /*  end of program    */
```

FIGURE C-1. Computer program for a Fourier transform.

i	A	B
0	1000	-1000
1	866	-866
2	500	-500
3	0.001	0.001
4	-500	500
5	-866	866
6	-1000	1000
7	-866	866
8	-500	500
9	0.001	0.001
10	500	-500
11	866	-866
12	1000	-1000

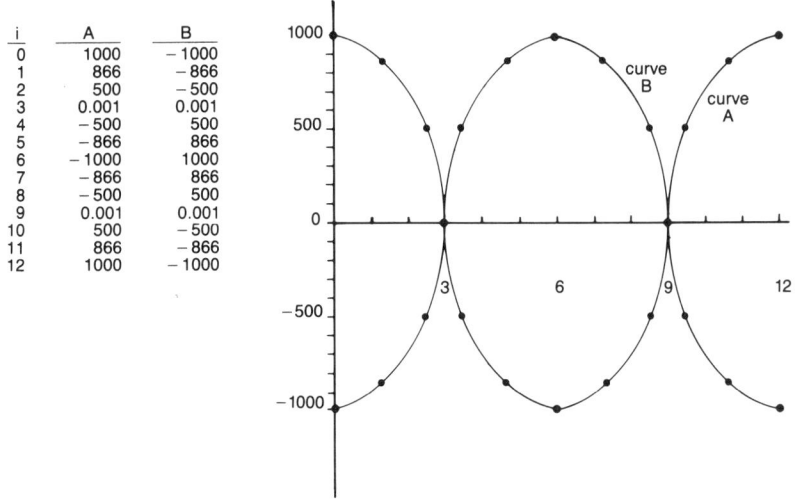

FIGURE C-2 Cosine curves (curves A and B) are 1800 out of phase with each other.

APPENDIX

D

The following are color illustrations of images shown in Chapters 8 and 9.

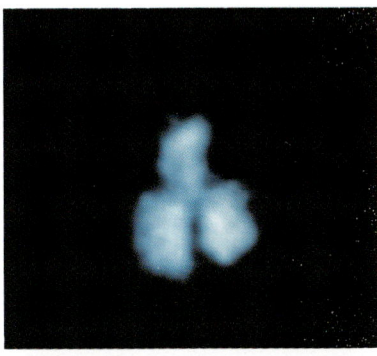
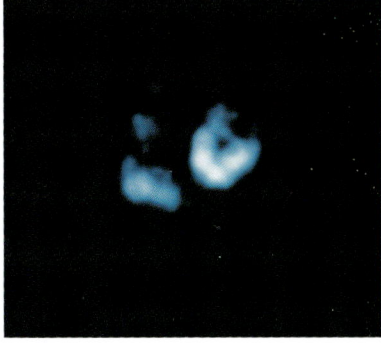
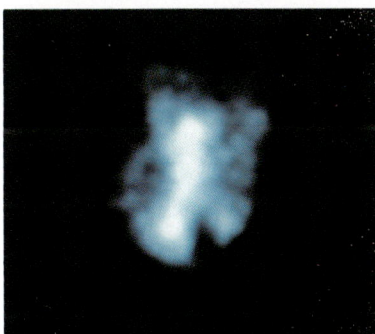

FIGURE 8-11 The stroke-volume image is obtained by subtracting the systolic image from the diastolic image.

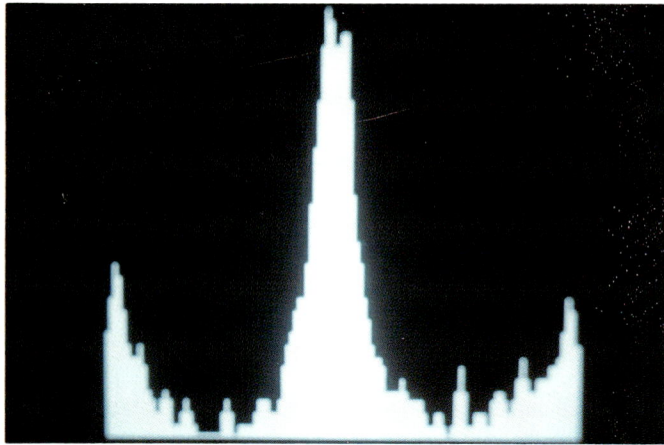

FIGURE 8-14 When the phase angles of all pixels within the heart are plotted, we obtain a histogram with two peaks. The peak near the 0° corresponds to the ventricles, and the 180° peak corresponds to the atria.

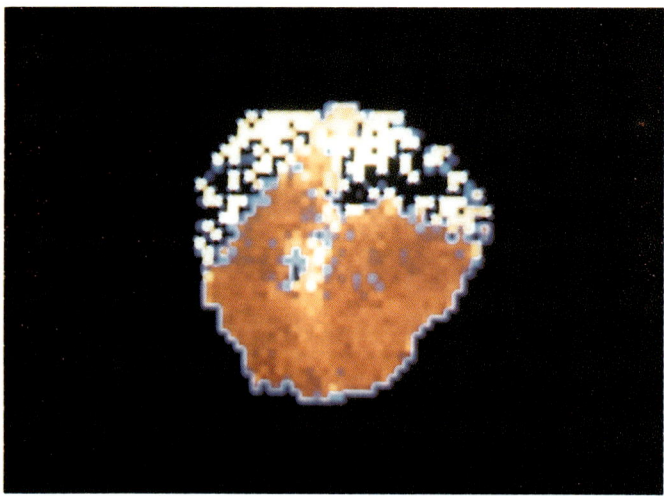

FIGURE 8-15 A phase image displays each pixel in a color corresponding to its phase angle. An abnormal region may appear in a color distinctly different from that of its neighbor.

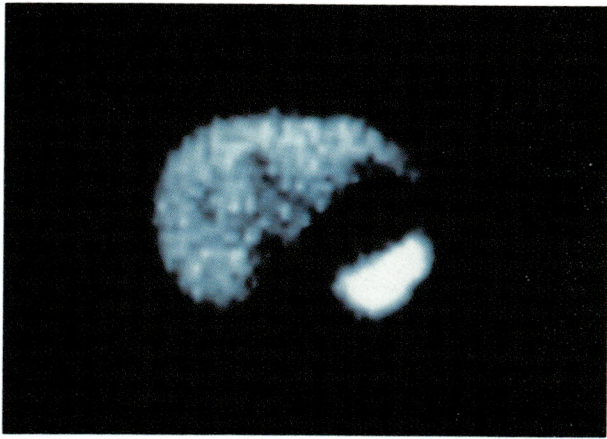

FIGURE 9-12 Images reconstructed with a ramp filter are unsatisfactory with much high frequency noise.

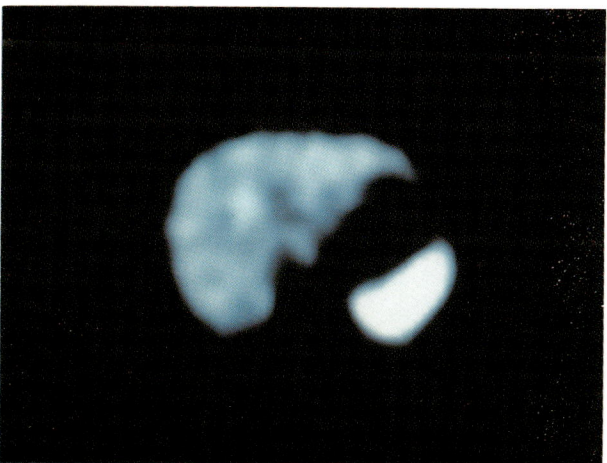

FIGURE 9-15 An image reconstructed with the Butterworth filter in Figure 9-14. Compared with images reconstructed with a ramp filter, the high-frequency noise was removed at the expense of reduced resolution.

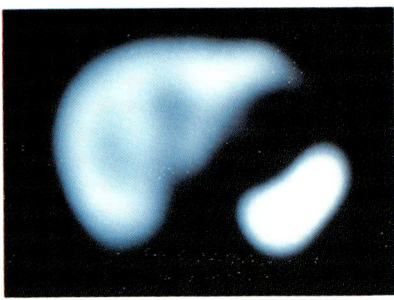 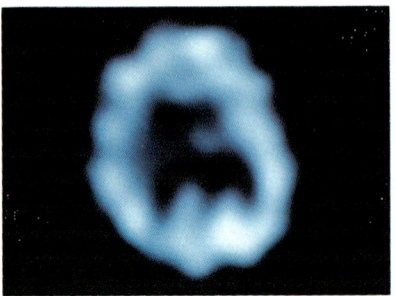

FIGURE 9-17 The Butterworth filter in Figure 9-16 produces an oversmoothed transfer image and is not useful clinically.

FIGURE 9-18 Due to an abundance of noise from poor count statistics, the Butterworth filter in Figure 9-16 produced a satisfactory image of ^{123}I-labeled iodoamphetamine in the brain.

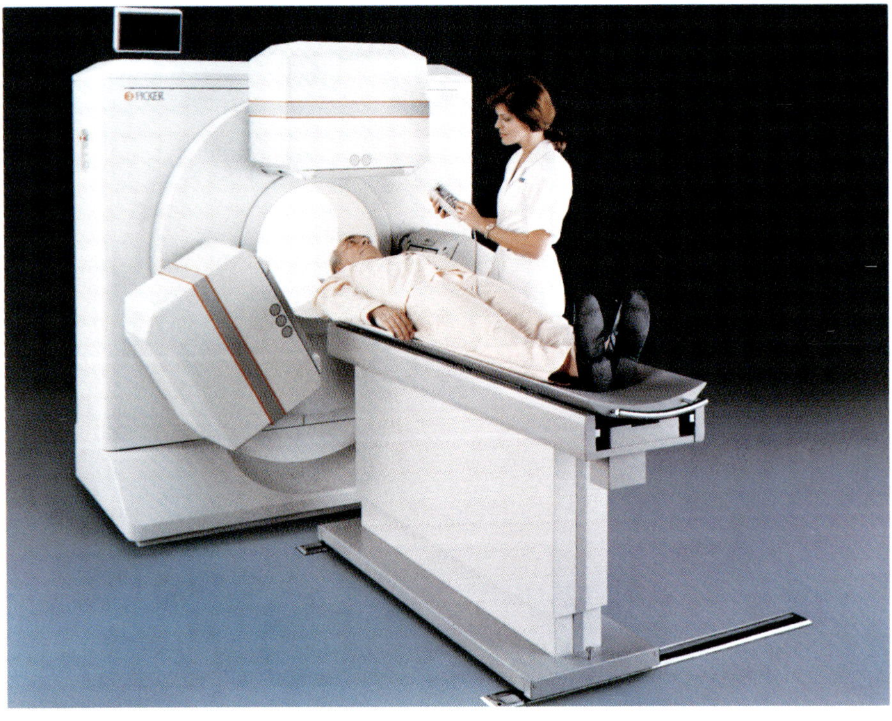

FIGURE 9-25 SPECT systems with three detectors will be able to collect more counts, hence higher image resolution, in the same imaging time as a single detector system (Reprinted courtesy of Picker, Inc.).

INDEX

Access arm, 24
Acoustic coupler, 45
Acquisition, 73
  parameters, 245
Acquisition matrix, 91
Activity
  profile, 110f, 111
  SPECT, 194, 195f
  -versus-time curve, 134, See also Time-activity curve
Ada, 81
ADC, See Analog-to-digital converter
Algorithms, 87
Aliasing, 208, 208f
Amplitude
  analysis, ejection fraction calculation by, 175-176
  modulation, 46, 47f
Amplitude image, 175
  analysis of, 175-176
Analog devices, 99
Analog electric voltage pulses, 48
Analog signal
  conversion to, 259-261
  differentiated from digital signal, 49, 49f
Analog-to-digital conversion (ADC), 48-50
Analog-to-digital converter (ADC, AC/DC), 43, 48-50, 88
  performance of, 261
  successive approximation of, 259-261
Angiography, contrast, 181
Angular sampling criteria, SPECT, 209-210
Application software, 68, 70f, 87
Architecture, computer, 5
  parallel, 6-7
Arithmetic and logic unit (ALU), of CPU, 3
Arithmetic operation, 8, 192
  simple point, 113
Array processor, 192-193
Arrhythmias, artifacts from, 153-155f
Artifacts
  aliases, 208
  from arrhythmias, 153-155f
  from delayed gating, 158

  hot rim, 210
  starburst, 195, 197f, 197
Assembler, 76
Assembly, 76
Assembly language, 75-77
  advantages of, 77
  portable, 83
  routines in, 77
  translation into machine language, 76
Asymmetric window, use of, 215
Asynchronous methods of transmission, 48
Atrium, See also Left atrium pixels in,
  phase angle of, 173
Attenuation, correction methods, 214
Attenuation coefficient, 214
^{195m}Au/^{195m}Hg generator, 182
Audio tones, 45
Automatic edge detection methods, 129
Averaging, 102
Axis of rotation, 223

Background, 73, 134
Background subtraction, 113-114, 128-129
  gray scale threshold in, 119-120
  interpolated, 115-117
  scaling the pixel brightness, 119
Backprojection method, SPECT
  filtered, 193, 197-200
  simple, 193-197
Backup
  off-line, 21-22
  Winchester disks and, 26
Band-pass filter, function of, 112
Bandwidth, 58-60
Baseband method, for transporting data, 232, 233
BASIC (Beginner's All-purpose Symbolic Instruction Codes), 81-82
Batch mode, 71
Batch processing, 73, 81
Baud rate, 44
Beginner's All-purpose Symbolic Instruction Codes, See BASIC
Binary arithmetic, 8
Binary code, 43, 74, 75, 76
Binary digit, 8, See also Bit

Binary form, conversion to, 259-261
  decimal, 257
Binary point, 256
Binary signals, 45, 49f
Binary system, 256-257
Bit, 8-10, See also Byte
  core memory, 17-18
  memory for future, 18
  quantity processed, 10
  semiconductor memory, 15-16
  word and, 9, 10
Black and white monitor, See also
    Monochrome monitor
  displays on, 121
Blood, volume, change, during R-R
    interval, 171
Blood-pool studies cardiac
  data acquisition method, 147, 148-158,
    See also Data acquisition
  multiple-gated acquisition in, 150-152f
  equilibrium, 164
  gated, See Gated blood-pool studies
  requirements for, 246
Blurring pixel mask, 102
Body contour
  following method, 216
  measurement of, 213
Bolus, passage through left ventricle, 178
Boot, 71
Booting, 11, See also Bootstrapping
Bootstrapping, 11-12, 71
Broadband method, for transporting data,
    232, 233
Bubble, 34, 36
Buffer memory, 13-15, 155-158
  SPECT computers, 192
Buffered gated-beat acquisition,155-158
Bug, See also Debugging; error
  phase diagram and, 267-268
Bulk-storage device, 42
Bus network, computers in, 236-237
Butterworth window, 203-204
Byte, 8-10, 17, 93, See also Bit
  defined, 8
  for pixel formation, 93, 94
  word and, 9, 10
Byte-mode acquisition
  disadvantages of, 95
  versus word-mode acquisition, 93-95

C language, 82-83

Cable
  network
    coaxial, 230, 231-232
    fiber optics, 231-232, 232f
    parallel, 230, 231f
    telephone, 45
Cache memory, 12-13
  size of, 13
Camera, See Gamma camera
Cardiac contractility, assessment of,
  multiple-gated images for, 159
Cardiology, nuclear, 147, 187, See also
    Blood-pool studies
  data acquisition in, 148-158, See also
    Data acquisition
  first-pass cardiac studies, 97, 176-185,
    See also First-pass cardiac studies
  multiple-gated acquisition in, 97
  planar quantification of myocardial per-
    fusion, 185-187
  quantitative data analysis in, 164-176,
    See also Ejection fraction
Carrier sense multiple access method
  (CSMA), 237
Carrier wave, 46
  modulation of, 46-48
Cathode ray tube (CRT), 53, 88
  images recorded off, 60
  monochrone, 53f, 53-56
Central processing unit (CPU), 2-3, 19
  arithmetic and logic unit, 3
  control unit of, 3, 4, 6
  criteria for selection, 251-252
  function of, 11
  instruction codes, 74-75
  memory unit, See Memory; Memory
    unit
  operating system loaded into, 71
  performance rating of, 4-5
  parallel processing, 6-7
  reduced instruction setcomputers, 5-6
  R-R time interval measurement by,156,
    157
  SPECT computers, 192, 193
  speed of, 4
    buffer memory and, 13-15
    in time-sharing modes, 72
    in wait-state, 13
    word-length, 10-11
Character generator, 44
Chest radiographs, 240

INDEX 277

Circuits
  integrated, 5
  very large scale, 18
  on or off condition of, 15, 16
CISC, *See* Complex instruction set computers
Clinical processing protocol, 247
Clinical software package, 99
Clock, 4
Coaxial cable, 230-231
  data transmission through, 232-233
Cobalt-57 (^{57}Co) disk marker, 224
Cobalt-57 (^{57}Co) flood sources, 222, 223
COBOL (Common Business Oriented Languages), 78-79, 80
Codes, 67
  symbolic, 67
Cold defect, 89
Collimator channel, field of view of, 215-216
Color
  display, economics and esthetics of, 58
  selection of, 121-122
Color gun, intensity scale for, 121
Color monitors, 44, 54, 56-60, 122
  color translation table, 121-122
  compared to monochrome monitors, 58
  NTSC (National Television System Committee), 57
  resolution of, 58, 60, *See also* Resolution
  RGB (Red-Green-Blue), 57
Color scales, 250
Color translation table, 121-122
Command function, 70, 71
Common Business Oriented Languages, *See* COBOL
Communication linkage with computer, 45
  acoustic coupler as, 45
Communication networks, *See* Networks, communication
Compiled language, 85
Compiler, 84
Complex instruction set computers (CISC), 5
Composite video monitors, *See* NTSC color monitor
Compton-scattered photons, 213
  reduction of, 213-215
Computed tomography, single-photon emission, *See* Single-photon emission computed tomography

Computer
  architecture of, 5
  developments in, 18
  inefficient use of, 13
  selection of, criteria for, 243-244, 253-254
  hardware, 251-253
  image display, 250
  reliability and service support, 253
  software, 244-247, *See also* Software
  user friendliness measurement, 249
  user support, 248
  SPECT, 190, 191f, 191, 192-193
  start-up procedure, 11, *See also* Bootstrapping
Computer networking, *See* Network
Computer program, *See* Software
Computer system, basic structures of, 1-2, 18-19
  bit, 15-18, *See also* Bit
  central processing unit, 2-7, *See also* Central processing unit
Conservation of Ignorance, law of, 98
Contrast enhancement, 113, 129
Control unit, of central processing unit, function of, 3, 4, 6
Convolution filter, 102, 105
  function of, 107, 113
Convolution filtering, 107
  alternative methods of, *See* Fourier filter
Convolution kernel, 102, 104
  smoothing, 102
Core memory, 17-18
  disadvantages of, 18
Correction factors, matrix of, 221
Couch, patient support, 191
Count(s)
  background, subtracting of, 128-129, *See also* Background subtraction
  distribution, in input image, 104
  gamma camera, 87
    amplification of, 91
  gray scale, 128-129
  for image formation, 90, 91
  in list-mode acquisition, 148
  matrix dimension, doubled, 220
  in multiple-gated acquisition, 151
  normalization procedure, 159, 162-163
  pixel, 88, 95, 113
    maximum number of, 94
    overflow, 94
  in ray-sum, 197, 198f, 199

temporal smoothing and, 160-161
threshold, 128-129, 165
Count data, 99
for radionuclide image, 56
Count rate
Compton-scattered photons and, 214
computer capability, 245-246
Count statistics, 204
poor
images with, non-normalized gray scale assignments, 119
left ventricular, 165
CPU, See Central processing unit
CRT, See Cathode ray tube
"Crumbs," 10
Curve, generation and analysis of, 134-136, 145
data smoothing by curve fitting, 139-145
moving-average method, 136-138
weighted, 138-139
Curve data, smoothing of, 138-139
Curve derivative,
first, 129
second, 130f, 131-132
Curve fitting, data smoothing by, 139-145
Curve smoothing
eye-balling, 135-136
moving average methods, 136-138

Daisy wheel printers, 60-62
Data
accidental loss of, backup for, 21
acquisition, See Data acquisition
manipulation, 3
reformatting of, for first-pass cardiac studies, See First-pass cardiac studies, data reformatting for
smoothed, 137, 137f
smoothing, 136, See also Smoothing by curve fitting, 139-145
transmission of, 23
in networks, methods of, 232-233
Data acquisition
in blood-pool studies
artifacts from arrhythmias, 153-155f
buffered gated-beat acquisition, 155-158
list-mode acquisition, 148-149
multiple-gated acquisition, 150-152f
temporal resolution, 153

in first-pass cardiac studies, 177
methods of, 87-88
rate of, 246
Data communication, speed, in PACS, 239-240
Data fudging, 198f, 199
Data points, 136-137
Deadtime, 95
reduction of, 96
Debugging, 75
C program and, 82-83
phase diagram for, 267-268
Decay, radioactive, 222
Decimal counting, 256
Decimal system, 255
Decimal to binary conversion, 257
Decision-making functions, mathematical and logical, in Pascal, 80
Demagnetization, 33-34
Derivative algorithms, first and second, 165
Derivative curve
first, 129, 130f, 131
second, 130f, 131-132
zero of, 132
Details, 111
Detector
motion, non-circular, 215-218
scanner-based, 190
Diastolic image, 175
Digital computer, 99
Digital image storage system, in PACS, 238-239
Digital modulation, 46
Digital modulator, 46
Digital number systems
binary system, 256-257
decimal counting, 256
decimal system, 255
decimal to binary conversion, 257
Digital signal
changing of analog signal to, 48-50, See also Analog-to digital converter
differentiated from analog signal, 49, 49f
Direct access storage device, 21
Discrete Fourier transform (DFT), 263-264
phase diagram, 267-268
Discrete values, 49
Disk
dual-fixed removable, 25
floppy, 30-32

hard, 22, 27
memory addresses on, 22
optical, see Optical disk
Disk cartridge, 24
Disk drive
criteria for selection, 252
floppy, 31
hard, 31
magnetic tape, 21, 37-41, See also Magnetic tape drives
multi-platter, 24-25
malfunction in, 21
optical, 21-22
for SPECT computers, 192
Disk-emulation duties, 29
Disk marker, 224
Disk optimizers, 29
Disk pack, 25
Disk partitions, 27
Disk platter, Winchester, 26
Disk space, SPECT, 192
Disk storage device
criteria for selection, 252
magnetic, See Magnetic disk storage devices
Diskette, See Floppy disk
Display, criteria for selection, 252-253
Display controller, 14, 15, 56
Display memory, 14, 15
advantages of, 56
Display monitor, See Monitor
Display unit, 14
Distance, radiation intensity measured at, 142-144
Distance-weighted averages, pixel, 116
Distortion, 105
Dose administration, in first-pass cardiac studies, technique for, 177
Dot matrix printer, 61-63
fonts, styles and symbols available to, 62
Dot pitch, 58, 59
Double-density format, of floppy disk, 31
Drawing, light pen for, 51
Drum, of laser printer, 64
Dual-fixed removal disk, 25
Dust particle, 24
Dynamic frame, rapid, reformatting of, 180-181, 181f
Dynamic frame-mode acquisition, 95-97
multiple-gated acquisition, 150-152f

Dynamic heart study, data acquisition for, 151
Dyskinetic region, free ventricular wall, 170
ECG, See Electrocardiograph
Edge
detection, 131
automatic, 129
gradient method for, 131
enhancement, with Fourier filter, 107
sharp, 111
Edge-enhancement filters, 105-106f
Edge points, determination of, 132
Ejection fraction (EF), 127, 153
calculation of, 153
amplitude analysis, 175-176
by first-pass studies, 181-182
functional images, 167-170
left ventricular region of interest, 164-165
phase analysis, 170-175
volume curve, 165-167
Ejection rate, peak, 167
Electrical power, MOS memory and, 16
Electrical pulses, 87-88
Electrocardiogram (ECG), electrocardiograph
gated list-modedata, reformatting of, 178-179, 180f
gating devices, 158
R-R time interval, See R-R time interval
R-wave, See R-wave
signals, 150, 151
Electron beam, 54, 55f
color monitor vs. monochrome monitor, 58
intensity of, 56
Electron gun, 54
intensity of, color and, 121
voltage, 56
Electrostatics, 62
Ellipse, body as, 213
Elliptical orbit, 216
End-diastole (ED), 163
Equilibrium blood-pool studies, 164
Errors, 82, See also Bug, debugging on magnetic tape, 40
minimizing of, 40-41
SPECT, 220, 221
truncation, 95

Even parity, 40
Execute, 76
Exercise, graded, 182
Eye-balling, 135-136, 140
Fast Fourier transform (FFT), 267
Ferric oxide, 22
Ferrite core, 17
Fiber optics, data transmission via, 231-232, 232f
File, 27
  defragmentation, 27-29
  management, 70, 73
Filling rate, peak, 167
Filter(s)
  band-pass,112
  convolution, 102, 105, 107, 113
  edge-enhancement, 105-106f
  Fourier, 108-113
  fudge, 200
  optimal reconstruction, 204
  ramp, See Ramp filter
  smoothing, 100-105, 111-112
  spatial, 199
Filtered backprojection method, SPECT, 193, 197-200
Filtering
  convolution, 107
  Fourier, 107-108
  low-pass, 112
Fine details, 111
Firmware, ROM, 12
First-pass cardiac studies, 97, 176
  data acquisition technique, 177
  data reformatting for, 178
  of ECG gated list-mode data, 178-179, 189f
  intra-cardiac shunt detection, 182-185
  of non-ECG gated list-mode data, 179
  of rapid dynamic frames, 180-181, 181f
  ventricular function evaluations, 181-182
Flood correction matrix, pixels in, 222-223
Flood image, pixels in, 222
Flood phantom, 221
Floppy disk
  description of, 30-32
  double-density format, 31
  for micro-computers, 31-32
  single-density format, 31
Floppy disk drives, rotation speed of, 31
Flow kinetics, of radionuclide, 95
Flow study, acquisition of, phases of, 245
Foreground/background operation, 73
Formatting, 31
  magnetic disk for, 22-23
  of optical disks, 24
FORTRAN (FORmula TRANslation), 78, 79, 80
Fourier analysis, 108-109
  fundamentals of, 107-108
Fourier components, 266-267
Fourier filter(s), image, 108-113
Fourier filtering, 107-108
  understanding of, 107
Fourier mathematics, phase analysis, 170-175
Fourier techniques, convolution of, contrast enhancement in, 129
Fourier transform, 263-270
  discrete, 263-264, 267-268
  fast, 267
  inverse, 108, 266-267
  one-dimensional, 112
  two-dimensional, 112
Frame
  normalization, 162-163
  number of, 245
Frame buffer, 14, 15, 56, 96
Frame-mode acquisition, 88-93, 94, 148
  dynamic, 95-97, 150-152f
  multiple-gated, temporal resolution in, 153
Frame processing operations, 123
Framing rate, 54, 96, 245
Frequencies, unwanted, removal of, 107, 111-112
Frequency domain, 108
  image manipulation in, 112
  image transformation into, 107-108
  transforming of radionuclide to, from space domain, 109-110
Frequency modulation (FM), 46, 47f, 48
Frequency shift keying (FSK) technique, 48, See also Frequency modulation
Fudge filters, 200
Full-duplex modes, 48
Functional images, for ejection fraction calculation, 167-170

INDEX

Gallium, background counts in, 129
Gamma camera, 48
  analog-to-digital converter interfaced to, 50
  counts collected from, 87, 245, *See also* Count amplification of, 91
  data input to computer by, 148-149
  rectangular matrix, 245
  shutter speed, 151
  signals produced by, 88
  spatial resolution of, 149
  SPECT, 190, 191f, 191-192
    center of rotation, 223
    detectors, 220
    field uniformity, 221-223
    non-circular detector motion, 215-218
    orthogonality and centering, 226, 227f
    pixel size, 223-226
    quality assurance, 221
    radius of rotation, 216, 217f,
    scattered photons in, 213-215
  square matrix, 244, 245
  square mosaic, 88
  voltage pulse from, 49
Gamma function, 184
Gantry, 191
"Garbage in garbage out syndrome," 3
Gated-beat acquisition, buffered, 155-158
Gated blood-pool studies
  multiple, *See* Multiple gated blood-pool studies
  ventricular, 144-145, 145f
Gated list-mode data
  ECG, reformatting of, 178-179, 180f
  non-ECG, reformatting of, 179
Gating, delayed, artifacts from, 158
Gaussian function, 184
Geometric operations, 123-124
Gigabyte, 10
Gradient, 129
Graphical user interface (GUI), 252
Gray scales, for video image display, 117-121, 250
  exponential, 120, 121
  imposing a threshold on, 119-120
  linear, 117, 119
  logarithmic, 120-121
  non-normalized, 119

Half-duplex modes, 48
Hard disk, 22
  performance of, optimizing of, 27
Hard disk drives, 31
Hardware, 70f
  arithmetic, array processor, 192-193
  categories of, 1
  criteria for selection, 251-253
  defined, 67
  electronic interconnection of, 230
  image display system, 250
Head crash, 24
Heart studies, *See* Cardiology, nuclear
Heart wall
  free, dyskinetic region of, 170
  motion, assessment of, 151
    blood-pool images for, 163
    qualitative, 153
High frequency terms, 109, 111
High resolution images, display of, 54
Histogram plot of phase angle, 173-175
Hot rim artifacts, 210
Hot spot, 89, 90f
Hues, creation of, 57
Hypercube design, 6-7

I/O devices, *See* Input/output devices
Image
  acquisition methods, 87, *See also* Acquisition
    byte-mode versus word-mode acquisition, 93-95
    data acquisition, 87-88
    frame-mode acquisition, 88-93, 95-97
    multiple-gated and list-mode acquisition, 97
    SPECT, 191
  analysis
    qualitative, *See* qualitative image analysis
    quantitative, *See* Quantitative image analysis
  control, SPECT and, 189
  display, gray scales for, 117-121
  enhancement, 99-100
    convolution methods of, edge-enhancement filters, 100-106f
    defined, 99
    Fourier methods of, 107-113

filtered, 111
magnification, 124
manipulation processes, 159
minification, 124
process selected, 250
processing of, 7, See also Processing software for, 247
quality of, 250
reconstruction, SPECT, 192
resolution, 252, See also Resolution
smoothing, See also Smoothing with Fourier filters, 107
Image array, 88
Image display station, in PACS, 238
Image display system, 250
Image matrix, 88, 93
 pixels in, 88-90
Image noise, See Noise
Image smoothing filters, 100-105
Image storage systems, digital, 238-239
Impact printing techniques, 60
Ink-jet printers, 62, 64, 64f
Input devices
 acoustic couplers, 45
 analog-to-digital converters, 43, 48-50, 88, 261
 defined, 43
 keyboard terminals, 43-44, 67
 modems, 45, 46-48
Input image, 102
 count distribution in, 104
Input/output (I/O) devices, 13, 14f, 43
Input/output (I/O) functions, 70, 73
 pause for, 13, 14f
Instruction(s), 1-2
 number of, 5
 pipelining of, 5
Instruction sets, 3
Integrated circuits, 5
 size of, 5
Inter-connection schemes, computer, 234
 bus network, 236-237
 ring network, 234, 236
 star network, 234
Interlace, 54-55
Intermediate calculation, SPECT, 192
Interpolated background subtraction, 115-117
Interpreted language, 85
Interpreter, 84
Intra-cardiac shunts, detection of, for first-pass studies, 182-185

Inverse Fourier transform, 108, 266-267
Ischemic areas, thallium imaging of, 185, 186
Joystick, 43, 51, 52, 53
 analog-to-digital converter connected to, 50
 creating ROIs with, 127
Juke box, 34, 42

Key, 67
Keyboard, 43-44, 67
Keypad, numerical, 44
Kidneys, visualization of, 123

Language, See Machine language; Programming languages
Laser, for optical disk, 34, 35f, 36
Laser printers, 62, 63-64
 printing speed of, 63-64
Law of Conservation of Ignorance, 98
Least-square curve
 fitting criterion, 140-145
 non-linear, 145
Left atrium
 left ventricle ROI and, 175
 time-activity curve, 172-173
Left ventricle
 blood pool in, 163
 bolus passage through, 178
 edge, 165
 ejection fraction, See Ejection fraction
 phase histogram, 174
 region of interest, 175
 ejection fraction calculation by, 164-165
 time-activity curve, 172-173
Lesion volume, measurement of, 223
Letter quality printers, See also Daisy wheel printers
 printheads, 61-62
Light, 231-232
Light pens, 43, 50-51
Linear gray scale, 117
Linear sampling criteria, SPECT, 207-209
Linear least-squares curve fitting procedure, 140-145
List-mode acquisition, 97, 246
 in first-pass cardiac studies, 177
 in nuclear cardiology, 148-149
 advantages of, 150
 shortcoming of, 150

INDEX

List-mode data, gated, See Gated list-mode data
Load, defined, 76
Local area network (LAN), 230
  baseband, 233
  topology, 233-234, 235f
    bus network, 236-237
    ring network, 234, 236
    star network, 234
Logic functions, 3
  decision-making, in Pascal, 80
Long-word, 9
Loop circumference, in ring networks, 234, 236
Low-pass filtering process, 112
Lung
  tracer flow through, 183-184
  V/Q ratio of, 127

Machine language, 74-75
  assembly language translation into, 76
  writing a program in, 75
Magnetic cores, 17
Magnetic disk, 43
  use of, 22
Magnetic disk drives, 21
Magnetic disk storage devices, 22-24
  file defragmentation, 27-29
  floppy disks, 30-32
  future of, 32
    perpendicular recording, 32-34
  multi-platter disk drives, 24-25
  optimizing hard disk performance, 27
  RAM disk, 29-30
  Winchester disks, 26
Magnetic field, 32
Magnetic heads, 23-24, 32, 33f
  destruction of, 24
  head crash, 24
Magnetic tape, 21, 22, 42, 43
  data recording on, 40
  disk file transfer to, 29
  errors on, minimizing of, 40-41
  recording density of, increasing of, 39-40
Magnetic tape drives, 37-38
  reel-to-reel, 38-41
  tape cartridges, 41
Magnification, 124
Mainframe computers, Mips, 4
Mask
  blurring pixel, 102
  in nine-point smoothing, 102
  pixel, 104, 105-106
  shadow, 57, 58, 59
  sharpening, 105
Mass storage devices, 21-22, 42, 43
  direct access, 21
  on-line, 21
  magnetic disk, 22-34, See also Magnetic disk storage devices
  magnetic tape drives, 37-41, See also Magnetic tape drives
  optical disks, 34-37f, See also Optical disks
  sequential access, 21
Master program, 69, See also Operating system
Mathematical decision-making functions, in Pascal, 80
Mathematics, Fourier, 110-111, 170-175
Matrix
  linear sampling criteria, 207
  rectangular, 245
  square, 244, 245
  word, 192
Median smoothing, 105
Memory
  amount of, 245
  buffer, 13-15, 155-158, 192
  cache, 12-13
  core, 17-18
  CPU, 21, 29, 22, 251-252
  display, 14, 15, 56
  future of, 18
  location, 7
  random access, See Random access memory
  read-only, 11-12, 71
  semiconductor, 15-16
  virtual, 22
  word-length and, 10
Memory address, 7, 8, 10
Memory chip, number of bits in, 15
Memory element, 7
Memory unit, 2, 7-8, 10, See also Memory
  bits and bytes, 8-10
  costs related to, 8
  word-length, 10-11
Metal oxidative semiconductors (MOS), memories, 15-16, 17
  advantage of, 16
  RAM disks, 29-30

speed of, 18
Mice, *See* Mouse
Micro-computers
 floppy disks, 31-32
 Mips, 4
Micro-processor
 32-bit, 18-19
 in Winchester disk drives, 26
Micro-switch, 15
Million instructions per second (Mips), 4, 6
Minification, 124
Mnemonics, 75-76
Modem, 45
 carrier wave, 46
 description of, 45-48
 information coded by, transmissionof, 48
Modulation, 46
Monitor, 14, 53
 character displays, colors of, 44
 color, *See* Color monitors
 criteria for selection, 252-253
 monochrome, 53f, 53-56, *See* Monochrome monitors
 multiple viewing, 238
Monochrome monitors, 53f, 53-56
 compared to color monitors, 58
 resolution of, 58, 59
Mosaic, 56
 square, 88
Mouse, 43, 51, 52
Moving average method, of curve smoothing, 136-138
 weighted, 138-139
Multi-platter disk drives, 24-25
Multiple-gated acquisition methods for cardiac studies artifacts, from arrhythmias, 153-155f
 phase analysis, 170-175
 frame-mode acquisition, temporal resolution in, 153
Multiple gated blood-pool studies, 97, 150-152
 analysis of, 158-159
 frame normalization, 162-163
 qualitative data analysis, 159-160
 temporal smoothing, 160-162
Multiplexing, 231
Multiplication factors, matrix of, 221
Multiplier, positional, 255

Myocardial imaging, interpolated background subtraction method, 115-117
Myocardial perfusion, planar quantification of, 185-187

NaI crystal, 148
NaI detectors, 190
Negative side lobes, 197, 199
Neighborhood-dependent point operation, background subtraction, 115
Neighborhood-independent point processing operation, 113
Network(s), 229
 communication, 230
 data transmission methods, 232-233
 network transmission medium, 230-232
 local area, 233-237, *See also* Local area network
 overview of PACS, 237-240
 wide area, 230
Network server, 234
Network transmission medium, 230-232
Node
 in bus network, 236
 in ring networks, 236
Noise
 defined, 100
 ramp filter and, 203
 reduction of, 135
 smoothing filters for, 100-105
 SPECT, 218-220
 statistical, 90
Non-impact printers, 60, 62
 ink-jet, 64
 laser, 63-64
 limitations of, 62-63
Non-linear least squares curve, 145
NTSC (National Television System Committee) color monitor, 58
Numbers, 8
 decimal, 255-257
Numeric keypad, 44
Nyquist cut-off frequency, 204
 defined, 201
 ramp filter below, 203
 stops at, 202-203
Nyquist sampling theorem, linear sampling theorem and, 208-209

Object program, 84
Octa-word, 9
Odd parity, 40
Off-line backup, 21-22
Older computers, framing rate in, 96
On-line mass storage devices, 21
Ones, 74, 75
Operating system (OS), 68-69, 70f
 file management, 73
 functions performed by, 69-70
 classification of, 70-71
 loading into CPU, 71
 real-time, 72-73
 time-sharing, 72
Optical disk, 34-37f, 42
 erasable, 42
 read/write, 36, 37f
 formatting of, 24
 juke box, 34
 WORM (Write Once Read Many), 34, 36
Optical disk drives, 21-22
Optimal reconstruction filter, 204
Organ
 boundaries, 111
 poorly defined, 128
 region of interest, See Region of interest
 volume, measurement of, 223
OS, See Operating system
Output device, See also Input/output device
 defined, 43
 image display monitors, 53-60, See also Monitors
 screen pointing devices, 50-53
Oversmoothing, 205

PACS, See Picture archival and communication system
Paradox image, 168, 170, 170f
Parallel architecture, hypercube design, 6-7
Parallel cable, network, 230, 231f
Parallel processing, 6-7, 193
Parathyroid glands, visualization of, 123
Parity
 even, 40
 odd, 40
Parity check, 40
Pascal, 80-81, 82

Patient information management components, of PACS, 239
Peak ejection rate, 167
Peak filling rate, 167
Perfusion, See Myocardial perfusion
Periodic function, 171
Peripheral devices, 13, 251
 mass storage, 43
Perpendicular recording, magnetic, 32-34
Phase analysis, for ejection fraction calculation, 170-173
 presentation of results, 173-175
Phase angle, 171-172, 264, 266
 histogram plot of, 173-175
Phase diagram, 267-268
Phase modulation, 46
Phosphors, 44, 54
 triads, 56
Photon(s), 87
 attenuation correction, 223
 in SPECT, 210-213
 Compton-scattered, 213
 reduction of, 213-215
 flux, 219
 low-energy, 213
Photon-linked images, 218
Photon-starved images, 218-219
Physiologic functions, evaluation of, 127
Picture archival and communication system (PACS), 229, 237, 240
 digital image storage system, 238-239
 functions performed by, 237
 image display station, 238
 patient information management, 239
 state-of-the art, problems with, 239-240
Pins, of dot matrix printer, 61
Pipelining, 5, 193
Pixel
 activity of, calculated, 212-213
 adjacent, contrast between, 105
 background, weighted, 117
 brightness, scaling of, 119
 counts in, 88, 95, 113, See also Counts
  overflow, 94
 depth of, 93, 93f
 in flood correction matrix, 222-223
 in flood image, 222
 formation of, bytes used for, 93, 94
 gray level assignment for, 117-121
 in image matrix, 88-90
 in image smoothing filters, 100-105

linear sampling criteria, 207-209
location, in list-mode acquisition, 148
noise level, 220
phase angle of, See also Phase angle
  histogram plot of, 173-174
  in phase analysis, 171
saturation, 94
size, SPECT measurement of, 223-226
statistical noise in, 90
storage capacity of, 93
time-activity curve, Fourier transform
  of, 171-172
value, true, 212
weight assigned to, 116
in word-mode acquisition, 94
Pixel-by-pixel translation, 114
Pixel array, 88
Pixel averages, 105
Pixel averaging, 105
Pixel mask, 104
  coefficients, 105-106
  convolution required for, time saving
    in, 106
PL/1 (Programming Language/One), 79,
  80
Planar images, conventional, 218
Planar quantification, of myocardial perfusion, 185-187
Point processing operations, 113
  background subtraction, 113-117
  color translation table, 121-122
  gray scales for video image display,
    117-121
Point source, SPECT, 199
Pointing, light pen for, 51
Pop-up window, 252
Portable assembly language, 83
Positional multiplier, 255
Post-processing technique, photon attenuation, 211-212
Printers, 60
  daisy wheel, 60-61
  dot matrix, 61-63
  ink-jet, 64
  laser, 62, 63-64
  non-impact, 62-63
  slow paper, buffer memory and, 13
Printheads, of letter quality printers,
  61-62
Printing techniques
  impact, 60
  non-impact, 60

Private-branch exchange (PBX) telephone
  system, 234
Processing, parallel, 6-7
Program, structure of, 80
Program execution function, 70
Programming language, 69
  "all-purpose," 79
  compiled, 85 high-level, 74
  Ada, 81
  BASIC, 81-82
  C, 82-83
  COBOL, 78-79
  features of, 77-78
  FORTRAN, 78
  implementation of, 83-85
  Pascal, 80-81
  PL/1, 79
  syntax, 77
  interpreted, 85
  low-level, 74
  assembly language, 75-77
  machine language, 74-75
  use of, 74
  One, See PL/1
Programming software, 68, See also
  Programming language
Projection image matrix, center of rotation in, 223
Prompt, 71
Pulse-height analyzer, window, scattered
  photons falling within, 213
Punched cards, 21

Q_p function, 184
Q_p/Q_s ratio, 127
Qsh function, 184
Quad-word, 9
Qualitative data analysis, in nuclear cardiology, 159-160
Qualitative image analysis, 99
  frame processing operations, 123
  geometric operations, 123-124
  image enhancement, 99-113, See also
    Image, enhancement
  point processing operations, 113-122,
    See also Point processing operations
Quality assurance
  in first-pass cardiac studies, 177
  SPECT, See Single-photon emission
    computed tomography, quality
    assurance

Quantitative data analysis, in nuclear
cardiology, 164, *See also* Ejection
fraction
amplitude analysis, 175-176
functional images, 167-170
left ventricular region of interest,
164-165
phase analysis, 170-175
volume curve, 165-167
Quantitative image analysis, 127, 145-146
creating ROIs, 128-134
curve generation and analysis, 134-145,
See also Curve, generation and
analysis

R-R time interval, 151-152, 180
arrhythmias and, 153-154, 154f
artifacts from delayed gating and, 157f,
158
blood volume changes during, 171
in buffered gated-beat acquisition, 156f,
156
in data reformatting in first-pass
studies, 178-179
variations in, 162
R-wave, 151, 152, 154, 156, 178
Radiation activity, plotting of, function of
time, 140, 141f, 142f
Radiation detection device, SPECT, 190,
190f
Radii, 186
Radioactivity profiles, SPECT, 190, 190f
Radionuclide, flow kinetics of, 95
Radionuclide image, *See also* Image count
data for, 56
Radius of rotation, gamma camera, 216,
217f
RAM, *See* Random access memory
Ramp filter
below Nyquist frequency, 203
SPECT, 200-207
Butterfield window, modified,
203-204
modification of, 201, 202f, 203
noise, reduction of, 203
transverse image in, 202-203
Random access memory (RAM), 11
buffer memory, 13-15
erasure of information from, 12
Random access memory (RAM) disk,
29-30 as staging buffer, 27
Random noise, 220

Rapid dynamic frames, reformatting of,
180-181, 181f
Raster, 53, 54, 55
bandwidth, 59-60
brightness of, 56
size and shape of, 58
Ray-sum, 194-195, 196f, 210
attenuation correction and, 211
Compton-scattered photons and,
213-214
counts distributed in, 197, 198f, 199
linear sample of, 207
Read-only memory (ROM), 11-12
instructions stored in, 71
Read/write
operation on cartridge tapes, 41
of floppy disks, 31
of hard disk, 31
in magnetic disk, 23-24
time spent on, 27
Read/write optical disk, erasable, 36, 37f
Real-time operating system, 72-73
Recirculation, 184
Reconstruction algorithm, photon attenuation correction factor incorporated in, 210
Reconstruction filter, optimal, 204
Recording
perpendicular, 32-34
redundant, 40
Recording head, magnetic, 32, 33f
Rectangular matrix, gamma camera, 245
Reduced-instruction set computers (RISC)
description of, 5-6
objective of, 5
workstations, 4
Redundant recording, 40
Reel-to-reel drives, 38-41
Region of interest (ROI), 127
in blood-pool studies, 163
creating of, 128-134
edge detection and, 129, 131
fixed method, volume curve generation
by, 166
variable method, volume curve generation by, 166
ventricle, *See* Ventricle
Regression analysis, 139-140
Reliability, 253
Renogram, 95
region of interest in, 128
Replace averaging, 105

Resolution, 252
  temporal, 151–152, 153
Respiration cycles, gating of, 151
RGB (Red-Green-Blue) color monitors, 57
Rhythm analysis, 171, *See also* Phase analysis
Right anterior oblique (RAO) view, 176
Right-to-use protocol, 233
Ring network, computers in, 234, 236
RISC, *See* Reduced-instruction set computers
ROI, *See* Region of interest
ROM, *See* Read-only memory
Rotation
  axis of, 223
  center of, 223
  radius of, 217, 217f
Routines, in assembly language, 77
Run, 71

Saline flush, dose administration, 177
Sampling criteria
  angular, 209–210
  linear, 207–209
Scale factor, 94
Scaling process, 95
Scanner-based detectors, for SPECT, 190
Screen pointing devices, 50
  light pens, 50–51
  mice, trackballs, and joysticks, 51–53
Screen refresh rate, 54
Sector numbers, floppy disks, 31
Self-demagnetization effect, 33–34
Semiconductor memory, 15–16
Sequential storage devices, 21
Serial image acquisition, 95
Serial mode acquisition, *See* List-mode acquisition
Serial transmission protocols, 234
  in networks, 233
Service support, 253
Shadow mask, 57
  color monitor resolution effects of, 58
  dot pitch, 58, 59
Sharp edges, 111
Sharpening mask, 105
Shunts, intra-cardiac, detection of, 182–185
Single-beat length selection method, 157
Single-density format, of floppy disk, 31

Single-photon emission computed tomography (SPECT), 6, 189
  image quality, physical factors affecting, 207
    angular sampling criteria, 209–210
    Compton-scattered photons, 213–215
    image noise, 218–220
    linear sampling criteria, 207–209
    non-circular detector motion, 215–218
    photon attenuation correction, 210–213
  instrumentation-system description, 190–193
    computer system, 192–193
  mathematics of transverse image reconstruction, 193
    filtered backprojection method, 197–200
    ramp filter, 200–207
    simple backprojection method, 193–197
  quality assurance, 220–221
    camera field uniformity, 221–223
    center of rotation, 223
    orthogonality and centering, 226, 227f
    pixel size, 223–226
Sinusoidal curves, 172
Slave program, 69, *See also* Operating system
Slope, 129
Small organ, spatial resolution of, increasing of, 91
Smooth, three-point, 136
Smoothed data, 137, 137f
Smoothing
  by curve fitting, 139–145
  five-point, 137, 137f, 138
  nine-point, 134
  oversmoothing, 205
  purpose of, 160
  spatial, 159
  temporal, 159, 160–162
  wrapped around technique, 161
Smoothing filter, 100–105, 111–112
  median smoothing in, 105
  nine-point, 100–102
  replace averaging in, 105
Smoothing kernel, 102
  nine-point, 160

INDEX

Software, 67
 clinical software package, 99
 criteria for selection, 251, 253
 defined, 67
 expansion of, 251
 high-level computer programming languages, 77-85
 image display system, 250
 operating system, 69-74
 PACS, 239
 processing, 100. 247
 programming, 69
  low-level computer programming languages, 74-77
  system control, 68-69
  types of, 68-69
Software gate, 179
Sound frequencies, 45
Space domain, transformation of radionuclide from, into frequency domain, 109-110
Spatial filter, 199
Spatial resolution, 88, 149
 increasing of, 91
 limitation of, 91
Spatial smoothing, 159
SPECT, See Single-photon emission computed tomography
Speed
 of CPU, 4
 reduced instruction set computers and, 5
Spots, 36, 39
Square matrix, gamma camera, 244, 245
Square mosaic, 88
Square wave, construction of, 109, 109f
Staging buffer, 27
Stand-alone terminals, memory of, 44
Star network, computers in, 234
Starburst artifact, 195, 197f, 197
Start-up procedure, 11, See also Bootstrapping
Static acquisitions, 95
Storage devices, See also Mass storage devices
 module devices (SMD), 25, 25f, 26
Storage elements, 7
Stroke volume image, 168, 169f, 175
Structured programming, Pascal and, 80-81

Subtraction operation, background subtraction, 113-114
Super-mini computers, Mips, 4
Switch
 micro-electronic, 12
 micro-switch, 15
 On and Off, 74-75
Synchronous transmission, 48
Syntax, 77
System
 reliability, 253
 uptime, 253
System control software, 68
 operating system, 68-69
 utility programs, 68, 69
System utilities, See Utility programs
Systemic circulation, tracer flow through, 183-184
Systole, 173
Systolic image, 175

Tape cartridge drives, 41
Target-to-background ratio edge detection algorithms and, 134
 increasing of, 113-114
Tear-off menus, 252
Technetium-99m (^{99m}Tc), 214
 activity, quality assurance, 221
 dose administration, 177
 frame processing operations and, 123
 sequential first-pass studies using, 182
 source, intrinsic flood image of, 246
 ventricular blood-pool activity of, 165
Telephone cables, 45
Temporal resolution, 151-152, 153
Temporal smoothing, in nuclear cardiology, 159, 160-162
Terminals, stand-alone, 44
Thallium-201 (^{201}Tl), 185
 background counts in, 129
 myocardial perfusion images, 115
 cold spots in, 185-187
Three-dimensional image reconstruction, 6
Threshold count, 128-129, 165
Time
 finite length of, 148
 function of, radioactivity plotted as, 140, 141f, 142f

Time-activity curve
 in first-pass cardiac studies, 177
 Fourier transform of, 172
 pixel, 171-172
 in reformatting gated list-mode data, 179
 in reformatting rapid dynamic frames, 180-191
Time curve, activity versus, 134
Time markers, 178
Time-saving, 106
Time-sharing, 72, 82
Timing-mark, 148
Tissue attenuation, correction of, 211
Token ring-network, 236, *See also* Ring network
Tracer, flow, 134, 183-184
Track, misalignment of, 40
Trackballs, 43, 51
Transistors, 5
Transmission
 asynchronous, 48
 synchronous, 48
Transverse image, 202-203
Triads, 57
Truncation errors, 95

Uniformity correction matrix, 222
Uptime, 253
User friendliness, 82, 83
 measurement of, 249
User-hostile system, 249
User support, 248
Utility programs, 68, 69

V/Q ratio, 127
Vacuum tubes, 5
Ventricle, *See also* Left ventricle region of interest diastolic, 168
 in ejection fraction calculation, 166-167
 wall, *See* Heart wall
Ventricular function, assessment of, 181-182, *See also* Multiple gated blood-pool studies

Very large scale integrated (VLSL) circuits, 18
Video display, *See* Display
Video display screen, 44
Video display terminal (VDT), keyboard terminal, 43-44
Virtual memory, 22
Volume curve, 144
 for ejection fraction calculation, 165-167
 generation of, 166
von Neumann architecture, 2

Wait-state, 13
Weight, pixel, 116
Weighted moving-average method of curve smoothing, 138-139
Wide area network, (WAN), 230
Winchester disks, 26, 27
 in PACS, 238-239
 storage capacity of, 26
Window, pop-up, 252
Window function, ramp filter modification with, 201, 202f, 203
Wires, in network transmission medium, 230, 232
Word, computer, 8-9
 bits and bytes and, 9, 10
Word-length, 10-11
 longer, 10-11
Word matrices, 192
Word-mode acquisition, versus byte-mode acquisition, 93-95
WORM, *See* Write Once Read Many disk
Wrapped around technique, 161-162
Write function, *See* Read/write function
Write Once Read Many (WORM) disks, 34, 36

Yoke, 54, 55f

Zeroes, 74, 75
Zoomed mode, 91
Zooming, 91, 92f
 advantages of, 151